Baby Secrets

How to know your baby's needs

Jo Tantum and Barbara Want

MICHAEL JOSEPH
an imprint of
PENGUIN BOOKS

MICHAEL JOSEPH

Published by the Penguin Group
Penguin Books Ltd, 80 Strand, London WC2R 0RL, England
Penguin Group (USA) Inc., 375 Hudson Street, New York, New York 10014, USA
Penguin Group (Canada), 10 Alcorn Avenue, Toronto, Ontario, Canada M4V 3B2
(a division of Pearson Penguin Canada Inc.)
Penguin Ireland, 25 St Stephen's Green, Dublin 2, Ireland
(a division of Penguin Books Ltd)
Penguin Group (Australia), 250 Camberwell Road,
Camberwell, Victoria 3124, Australia (a division of Pearson Australia Group Pty Ltd)
Penguin Books India Pvt Ltd, 11 Community Centre,
Panchsheel Park, New Delhi – 110 017, India
Penguin Group (NZ), cnr Airborne and Rosedale Roads, Albany,
Auckland 1310, New Zealand (a division of Pearson New Zealand Ltd)
Penguin Books (South Africa) (Pty) Ltd, 24 Sturdee Avenue,
Rosebank 2196, South Africa

Penguin Books Ltd, Registered Offices: 80 Strand, London WC2R 0RL, England

www.penguin.com

First published 2005
7

Copyright © Jo Tantum and Barbara Want, 2005

The moral right of the authors has been asserted

Set in 11.5/14.75 pt Adobe Garamond
Typeset by Rowland Phototypesetting Ltd, Bury St Edmunds, Suffolk
Printed in Great Britain by Clays Ltd, St Ives plc

A CIP catalogue record for this book is available from the British Library

ISBN-13: 978-0-71-814709-9

Baby Secrets

Contents

Acknowledgements

I would like to dedicate the book to Hadleigh Elliott and Freya Poppy – Aunty Jo Jo loves you big up to the sky.

I would also like to make special acknowledgement to the following people:

To my Gran, who is no longer with us but I miss her every day. You would have been so proud of me, you always told me I could do anything. I just wish you were here to share it with me.

To the rest of my family, I am so lucky to have you. Especially my little Mummy, my amazing sister Nic and her husband, my Dad and his wife Kate, and my Aunty Cathryn, Uncle Keith, Laura and Marcus, for supporting me and believing in me every step of the way.

To all the wonderful families I have had the privilege of helping and for sharing their gorgeous babies with me. Special thanks to Mindy, Julian and their twins Sofie and LeLe. And to Annabel and Tony and their girls Lydia and Amaya, with whom I have become great friends over the years.

My long-suffering friend Sam Dance, who is always ready with a cup of coffee to listen and laugh. Even though after twenty-one years she still doesn't know how many sugars I have!

To my favourite place in the world, Adelaide, and all my friends there who are waiting patiently for my return. Especially to the Donato family, who took me under their wings.

Also to Tony, Ann and their girls, Hannah, Fiona and Kirsten, for giving me advice and helping me with so many things and for making me feel part of your family.

To Kate Adams at Penguin and David Miller at Rogers, Coleridge & White.

And to Barbara, who has helped me bring all my years of hard work and dedication to life in this book.

Jo Tantum
www.babysecretsltd.com

Thanks to David Miller at Rogers, Coleridge & White, and Kate Adams at Penguin, for taking this on. Also at Penguin, Georgina Atsiaris and Sarah Hulbert; and copy-editor Bela Cunha.

Thanks to the many people who offered advice or ideas, told their stories, or commented on the manuscript: Lidia Amorelli, Josephine Berry, Josh Claman, Susan Cohen, Margie Davies and Jane Denton at the Multiple Births Foundation, Julie Duncan, Kate Ferontelli, Robin Finlay, Helen Forbes and Gillian Smith at Tamba, the Twins and Multiple Births Association, Julia Fox, Mary Greenham, David Hass, Marion Hope, Helen Keenan, Jo Kessel, Jo Korn, Annabel Mackie, Sherry Mandel, Dan Murphy, Morag Preston, Ruth Reckitt at the Maternity Nurse Company, Amanda Rimmer, Nicola Ripon, Roger Sawyer, Rachel Schofield, Angie Shannon, Richard Tait, Kate Wolfsohn and many members of the Central London Twins Club – so many helped, but I cannot name them all.

Special thanks to those who somehow found time to go the extra mile for me in different ways: Jacki Claman, Ruth Dowsett, Mindy Glatt, Lucie Hass, Anita Kidgell, Lucinda McNeile.

The biggest thanks go to my twins Benedict and Joel, for giving me very little time to write but a huge amount of love and inspiration.

Finally – this is for my husband Nick, unequivocally.

Barbara Want

Introduction
The Best Beginning

Barbara

For me, becoming a parent was like discovering an extra drawer in a faithful old cupboard – full of magical wonders I never knew existed.

In my innocence I assumed that along with the baby – or, in my case, babies – would come those natural 'instincts', as reliable as mother's milk, telling me what to do next. But they were nowhere to be found. And that meant that when my boys cried (which they did frequently) I had no idea why, nor what to do about it. I didn't know how to feed or bath them, let alone how to avoid the path, trodden by so many others I knew, of round-the-clock feeding and sleepless nights stretching ahead across the months. And years . . .

I felt the stirrings of panic. Why hadn't the hospital given me an instruction manual along with the welcome pack? Was I capable of organizing this new life, in particular without sleep?

And then I met Jo.

Jo's understanding of babies, not to mention parents' need for reassurance and guidance, is second to none. She made promises I dared not believe but badly needed to hear. She said she would instil in me the confidence to understand my babies' needs and how to meet them. She promised order where chaos loomed. She told me my boys would thrive on this and soon be sleeping through the night.

I'm glad I believed her; she delivered on everything.

Jo's methods are not rocket science. They are straightforward and *really easy for any parent to follow*. She doesn't have a magic wand. But her methods work; they are flexible, kind to babies and very kind to their poor frazzled parents.

My boys loved the routines Jo showed us, and we slipped into them easily. I began to enjoy looking after two new babies, I got some control back over my life and we all loved the fact that the boys slept through the night at three months – and still do.

It was while Jo and I were sitting down over one of our many cups of tea talking about the wonders of routines and sleep that we came up with the idea for *Baby Secrets*. Between us we felt we could offer a unique combination: an expert in babycare and a parent who had tested out her methods.

We will help you decide what to buy (and what to avoid) before your baby arrives, and give you guidance on what to do in the first few days after your baby is born. You will find advice on getting your baby into a feeding routine once you – and he – are ready to embark on one, and there is a step-by-step guide towards the Holy Grail of parenting: getting your baby to sleep through the night. And because things don't always go smoothly, the book offers solutions to the difficulties every parent encounters along the way. Parents worry endlessly about their babies' health so there is a quick guide to common baby ailments, as well as some of the (sometimes embarrassing) ailments that afflict a mum after she's given birth. We've included a chapter on twins and some tips on how to help older siblings cope with a new arrival, advice on travelling with a baby and a few ideas on where to look for help with your baby, if you need to.

Most of it is common sense, but common sense is what

parents need. They also need faith. We want to share that
faith – with you.

Jo

I was fourteen when my cousin Laura was born; she was
gorgeous and I was hooked. I spent all my spare time – and
all my school holidays – with her, changing her nappy,
bathing her and begging to feed her. When her brother
Marcus arrived, I did the same. I soon realized what I wanted
to do in my life – I wanted to take care of babies. On the
childcare courses that followed I flew through the exams,
almost without trying; the answers seemed to come
instinctively. *I loved* the placements I did with babies and
the babies seemed to love me too.

After qualifying with my NNEB I worked in nurseries
and baby units before getting my first job as a maternity
nurse for newborn twins. I started by observing their
sleeping and feeding patterns and then used the information
to work out a routine for them. The sense of satisfaction I
felt as the babies slipped happily into it was amazing – and
even greater was the sense of achievement I felt when I got
them to sleep through the night. Their mother was
overjoyed too and I realized I had found my vocation . . .

I've never looked back. I've cared for many babies (and
their parents) over the years and it is still my passion. It
never ceases to amaze me though how such a tiny creature
can cause such mayhem – and so quickly; a household
that is organized and calm can descend into chaos in days.
The biggest mistake parents make is to try a hundred and
one different things in the hope that one of them will keep

the baby happy – or asleep. Sadly, this usually ends up confusing the baby and can make him frantic with frustration.

I understand what a daunting task it can be for parents to look after a baby, not to mention the huge responsibility they feel. So what I show them is done with sympathy and understanding. My job is to give them the confidence and skills they need both to care for their baby and to understand him. Once you know his needs – whether it's milk, sleep or a cuddle – you are on the way to having a happy baby and to being a confident and happy parent.

You can do this with my straightforward plan. It has two main aims: first, to get a baby into a feeding routine because once he is in a routine it is much easier to work out what he needs and why he is crying. My routines are based on babies' natural feeding and sleeping patterns, but because I know that all babies are different I ask parents to keep a log of their baby's patterns and use this to find the best routine for him. The second aim is to get a baby sleeping through the night at an early age. A baby who sleeps well is healthier and happier. (And so are his mum and dad . . .)

I always say to parents that if they stick to the plan for seven days they will see results and I give them a one hundred per cent guarantee that it will work. Many parents think I am a miracle worker, but all I have done is tried many techniques over the years and discovered the secret of which ones work best. I am so pleased that I can now pass all my secrets on to you.

Throughout the book babies are referred to as 'he' for ease, with the exception of the problem-solving chapters where both 'he' and 'she' are used. 'Newborns' are babies up to the age of about four weeks.

1.

The Secret to Being Prepared

'If you are a first-time parent and don't know the difference between a sleepsuit and a babygro, or a buggy and a pushchair (and you're too embarrassed to ask what a breast pump is), we promise you are not alone.

'So many people go into parenthood unsure of what they really need . . . and too often buy things they don't. Overenthusiastic shop assistants have an uncanny knack of persuading expectant parents to part with money for things they don't want, don't understand or have no room for. Wherever you do your shopping and whatever you decide to buy, do your research beforehand: ask friends for recommendations and try out their equipment. And keep an eye out for the latest products. This is a booming business and things change constantly.

'If you are reading this before your baby arrives and aren't sure what you need, we hope this chapter will help you to narrow down the essentials, and avoid the non-essentials.'
Barbara and Jo

Clothes

It's easy to get carried away with newborn outfits, and even if you don't, your friends may. Since babies grow out of newborn clothes in as little as a couple of weeks, stick to the minimum. Six sleepsuits/ babygros (all-in-one outfits with long sleeves and enclosed feet, usually poppered at the front) and six vests for daytime wear in summer or for underwear in winter should be enough, along with a couple of cardigans and a warm coat for cold weather.

Tumble drier

Baby washing piles up quickly and a tumble drier is one of the most useful pieces of equipment you can get.

Nappies

For parents worried about the environment or the prospect of spending hundreds of pounds on disposable nappies, there is an enormous choice of cloth alternatives. The plastic pants and bulky safety pins of our parents' generation are no more: today's cloth nappies fasten with plastic grips, poppers or Velcro and have a washable (or disposable) lining which is changed when the nappy is wet or dirty. The nappies are washed every few days and don't need to be soaked beforehand – so there are none of the smells associated with nappy buckets. You could even use a nappy-laundering service, which takes away your dirty nappies, launders them and delivers them back to your door.

Using cloth rather than disposable nappies can, according to enthusiasts, save you as much as £1,000. If you can't face the cloth option but your environmental conscience is still pricked, there are environmentally friendly disposables available (at a premium).

When using disposables you need not be restricted to branded. Most supermarkets do their own cheaper versions which are usually an excellent choice. One option is to use branded nappies at night, as they may have slightly better absorption over longer spells, and less expensive brands during the day.

Nappy bin

A specially designed nappy bin for disposables may not be more convenient than a standard bin with lid and a pack of fragranced nappy sacks. Nappy bins fill quickly and replacement cartridges are expensive.

Rocker chair

This is an item that parents sometimes overlook but is really worth getting and spending extra money on if you can; choose a well padded one with a tilt adjustment. At its lowest level it must lie flat so you can use it for your baby's naps.

A rocker chair is a great place for a baby to while away the hours: you can place an activity arch over the top to amuse him or tilt it so he can sit and watch you. The chair will also be useful when you wean your baby on to solids until such time as he is ready to support himself in a high chair.

Breast pump/Expressing machine

Many breastfeeding mums find a breast pump a godsend. Expressing can prevent engorgement, help to build up your milk supply and provide breastmilk for bottle feeds. Electric expressing machines pump both breasts at once and though bulkier and noisier than manual pumps, they seem to be more popular; you can buy or rent them and suppliers usually deliver overnight.

Bottles

Wide-necked bottles really do seem to reduce wind and colic as the manufacturers claim, and the wide necks also simplify the task of scooping in milk powder. Six bottles should be enough. If you are using bottles from the beginning check you have newborn teats, as most bottles are sold with second-stage teats. Stick to the larger 9oz bottles; the smaller ones will get only a few weeks' use.

Small or premature babies may find it hard to suck on silicone teats; use latex.

If time is of the essence you could splash out on a travel system with pre-sterilized disposable bags that will save you washing up and sterilizing.

Don't forget a bottle- and teat-brush for cleaning.

Sterilizers

Your options are:

- A bucket for rather foul-smelling sterilizing solution made from water and sterilizing tablets and in which bottles have to be immersed for a minimum of half an hour
- An electric steam sterilizer
- A microwave sterilizer, which is quick to use, the only disadvantage being that most only take four bottles at a time
- Sterilizing bags (plastic bags into which you place bottles, water and a sterilizing tablet and then seal tight before heating in the microwave). They're convenient but the chemical-infused water can take its toll on your hands
- Sterilizer-bottles that can be sterilized directly in a microwave.

Jug for formula

Making up formula in advance saves time. It can be stored for up to twenty-four hours in the fridge, preferably in a jug with a seal-tight lid and pouring facility; or use milk powder travel dispensers to store pre-measured amounts of powder so that milk can be made up quickly when you need it. (An alternative is to use cartons of ready-made formula.)

Changing area

If your baby is going to sleep upstairs you will save time and energy by having a second changing area downstairs. If space is at a premium get a pull-down changing station which attaches to the wall.

Whenever you change your baby take care not to leave him unattended. Paediatric Accident and Emergency departments treat more babies for falls off mats than for almost any other accident. Parents don't always realize how mobile a baby can be.

Toys

Play time is an important part of your baby's day. Even tiny babies absorb and process information, and need to be stimulated and entertained.

A baby's eyesight does not mature fully until around eight months (when his eyes will also be close to their final colour). Newborns can focus no further than six to eight inches which, conveniently, means mum's or dad's face is in sight whenever baby is being held. Babies love eye-to-eye contact.

Babies can see colours from birth, but shapes in high contrast colours like black, white and red are the easiest to see at the start. Save cute-looking pastels until your baby is at least four months old.

Try these forms of entertainment:

- Black, white and red toys made specially for young babies
- Black and white pictures with strong images, or black, white and red fabric books (you can even use magazine photos or create some pictures yourself)

- An activity mat – a padded mat with an arch of brightly coloured toys hung over the top
- A play arch with dangling toys, which you can move to wherever your baby is lying
- Lullabies or classical music (you can buy baby-friendly classical selections). Classical music *may* help to stimulate a baby's brain (the so-called 'Mozart effect')
- Baby videos.

'Should I allow my baby to watch television? This is controversial territory.

'The view of some recent American research was certainly not. Children under two who did so were at risk of attention deficit disorders. But television producers have realized there is a gap in the market for "educational television" for babies, claiming that their videos "develop the cognitive processes of the brain" and "maximize and lengthen a baby's attention span".'

'I can only say that when they were little my boys watched a "Baby Mozart" video from the *Baby Einstein* series at least once a day. They loved the shapes, colours and music and it calmed them if they were fretting. I certainly don't think it did them any harm, although it's harder to judge whether it did any long-term good. At least it gave me a break, which is why I would recommend it.'

Barbara

For bathtime

Your baby's first baths could be in a small plastic baby bath, either free-standing or designed to be propped on top of your own bath. You can also use a reclining bath seat which will be useful until your baby can sit up unaided. Support sponges which float on the surface of the water can leave a baby chilly. He needs to get accustomed to the sensation of being *in* the water.

You will also need:

- A baby sponge
- Cotton wool to wipe your baby's eyes
- A couple of hooded towels.

And you might want a thermometer for the bath water.

Think twice before buying baby bath products such as shampoo or bubble bath; if your baby has sensitive skin they might cause a reaction. You could use Oilatum oil instead or baby products which are hypoallergenic.

For bedtime

Moses basket

A moses basket will last your baby around six to twelve weeks. You could bypass it and put your baby in his cot from the beginning, swaddling him to make him feel secure.

Cot or cot-bed?

This is a matter of personal preference. It may depend on how much space you have, and whether you're hoping to have more children who can take over a cot as their older sibling moves to a bed. A cot-bed should last until your child is about five. Choose a mattress that is firm and the very best you can afford.

The cot should not be positioned next to a radiator as over-heating is very dangerous; nor should it be under a window. If you are worried about temperature fluctuations, you could get a thermostatically controlled free-standing radiator for your baby's room.

Cot bumper

Cot bumpers provide padding round the end of the cot and should be tucked in firmly behind the mattress. Some parents avoid them for fear their baby will get his head stuck underneath, but research has shown that cot bumpers don't pose a risk. If the strings are long, cut them short.

Cot toys

Be wary of large stuffed toys as they can cover a baby's face. Bright objects or wall stickers round the cot are not a great idea; a cot is a place for rest, relaxation and sleep, rather than stimulation.

Cot mobile

The display cots in shops invariably have mobiles hanging above them and you might be forgiven for assuming that a mobile helps a baby to sleep. In fact, mobiles are best restricted to daytime use, particularly the morning when they can signal the start of the day.

Slumber Bear

'A Slumber Bear is an invaluable aid to teaching a baby to sleep at night and I try to persuade every parent I work with to get one. Slumber Bears house a small box with a recording of the sounds heard inside the womb: to you and me this is more like the gentle rumble of waves on a beach. The recording is triggered by the cries of an unsettled baby or by a gentle tap. I find it has a soothing effect on babies and helps them to resettle themselves to sleep when they wake in the night. Ideally, it should be used from newborn or from a few weeks after a baby is born. Some babies love their Slumber Bears so much they are still attached to them when they are three or four years old.'
Jo

Alternatives to a Slumber Bear are lullaby soothers which, in addition to lullabies, play calming nature sounds. Or you could choose to play a CD to lull your baby, but make sure all the tracks are restful. Avoid soothers with projected lighting: babies need to sleep and the equivalent of disco lights flashing round the ceiling will not help. Whatever you choose, make sure it is soothing and stick to the same sound every night.

Dark curtains or blackout blinds

Dark curtains with blackout lining or blackout blinds are invaluable in helping a baby to understand the difference between day and night and to learn to sleep well. Light seeping through curtains or over the curtain rail can startle a baby and wake him early, messing up your plans to get him to sleep through. You can get blackout blinds from department stores, or a specialist company can fit them.

One reason parents balk at the idea of blackout blinds is that when they travel and find themselves in a room without them, their baby wakes at the very first sign of light because he has got used to the dark. But all it takes is a sheet of blackout material or a dustbin bag, some sticky tape or pins, and you can create darkness wherever you are.

Once your baby is older and has learned to sleep well at night, you can relax about creating total darkness all the time.

Monitor

A monitor with a rechargeable portable parent unit is worth the premium in savings on batteries alone. The snag is that your baby's sounds, or even your own conversations, *may* be heard by any neighbours who have similar monitors. The more expensive models boast of having their own digital frequencies which can't be intercepted.

Some parents go so far as to have a sensor pad in their baby's cot: an alarm is activated if the baby stops moving for more than a certain length of time. These units can make parents overanxious as they are liable to sound for no reason, and there is no evidence that they reduce the risk of cot death.

Changing mat

This needs to be laid on a solid flat surface (maybe on top of a chest of drawers). Remember never to leave a baby unattended on a changing mat.

You will also need:

■ Wipes, but use cotton wool and water on your baby's bottom until he is at least two weeks old

- Cotton wool
- A small bowl for water to dip the cotton wool in
- Baby bath toys (such as baby bath books)
- Aqueous cream to moisturize your baby's skin (but be careful not to use it if your baby develops eczema as it may irritate the skin)
- A massage oil: you could use aqueous cream, grapeseed oil or specially prepared baby massage oil
- An antiseptic barrier cream or a soothing cream for nappy rash
- A mattress protector
- A couple of sheets, preferably cotton and fitted, for ease
- A couple of lightweight cotton sheets for swaddling (you could use pram sheets)
- A couple of blankets
- A sleeping bag. You can use a sleeping bag once your baby reaches about six weeks and no longer needs to be swaddled. Babies often sleep better in a sleeping bag: it can't be kicked off in the night and leave a baby uncovered
- A pack of muslins. These have many uses, from placing on your shoulder to catch regurgitated milk, to placing under your baby's head in his cot to save you having to change the sheets every time he is sick (tuck it in securely at the edges)
- A dimmer switch so you can keep the lights low when your baby is going to bed, and when you feed him in the middle of the night
- A baby thermometer: a digital ear thermometer is easy to use and worth spending money on
- A couple of dummies: the most convenient are those with covers to keep them clean and sterile (see pp. 38–9 for a discussion on dummies)
- Baby nail scissors.

For getting out of the house

A baby carrier

The Babybjorn is popular, but is at the top end of the market and with a price to match. Other manufacturers make similar carriers. Choose one that is well padded.

'Baby nests' (like slings) replicate the way babies are carried in nomadic or developing cultures, but, although they may settle an uneasy baby quickly, they may not provide great support for a baby's back. Nor are they as well padded and protected as carriers.

Pram, pushchair or buggy?

Think hard before buying a pram; your baby will want to sit up after about three months and you may no longer need it. It might be better to use a pushchair from birth, but be warned that, although many pushchairs are described as being suitable for new-borns, *if they do not go flat they are not suitable*. Babies, especially newborns, *must* be able to lie flat (or very slightly raised in a rocker chair) for most of their waking hours. This means that the truly lightweight buggies that don't lie flat and don't have much protective padding are suitable only for babies over six months.

Pushchairs need to have a five-point harness to comply with safety regulations.

Three-wheeler pushchairs (often known as all-terrain push-chairs) are easier to manoeuvre but can be bulkier than four-wheelers, as well as heavier and harder to collapse. Not all three-wheelers have a swivel front wheel as they are designed to be used over rough ground; if you are more likely to be pushing yours round a supermarket than an all-terrain environment this can be a drawback. Some three-wheelers have swivel wheels that can be locked if needed.

Should you get a travel system? These are popular but pricey. A travel system consists of a car seat which can be clipped on to a pushchair base to form a pram and later a pushchair, as well as on to a base in the car, saving you the trouble of lifting your baby in and out of different seats. The problem is that because they are so convenient, babies sometimes spend too much time in them. A baby under six months should not sit upright for more than two hours at a time; his bones are growing and it could be bad for his spine.

If you have an older toddler you might want a double buggy (see p. 226 in twins chapter) or you could try a buggy board.

Car seat

Be guided by ease of handling as you will probably use this seat to carry your baby to and from the car. You need a head-hugger for a newborn baby or his head will roll. A car seat should not be bought second-hand as it may have been involved in an accident and no longer be safe.

Changing bag

A specially designed changing bag will usually have a compartment to keep bottles warm, but you can survive without anything state-of-the-art; an ordinary mini-rucksack can do the job.

Inessentials and luxuries

Think carefully before buying a swinging crib – it may look appealing in the shop, but you will use it only for a few weeks. Your baby can nap in a rocker chair during the day and doesn't need to be rocked at night (or he will get used to the luxury and want it every night).

A night light isn't necessary. Babies are comforted by the dark as it reminds them of the months they spent in the womb.

Changing stations are appealing but not essential. A flat surface big enough for a changing mat is fine; an ordinary chest of drawers will have a longer shelf-life.

Electric bottle warmers are a luxury. Milk can be easily warmed in a bowl of hot water, or you can offer milk at room temperature (but be sure to take the chill off if it has come out of the fridge).

Breastfeeding 'gliding chairs' are lovely but expensive and bulky. An ordinary chair with good back support and that you can pad out with cushions or pillows is fine.

Battery-operated swinging baby chairs divide parents: some see them as a life-saver, others as an unnecessary luxury.

Nappy stackers keep nappies tidy but are not the only way to do so.

Sheepskin rugs are great for babies to snuggle on, but they must not sleep on them.

Sheepskin buggy liners can be used in winter and summer, when the natural fibres absorb moisture from the skin.

Organization

It may not be rocket science, but when you plan your baby's sleeping area some of these simple tips might be helpful:

- Have the changing area as near to the cot as you can so you don't need to carry your baby round the room at night.
- Find space for a small bowl, cotton wool and cream next to the changing mat or on a shelf directly above so it is within reach.
- Put nappies in the top drawer of the unit/chest of drawers

on which you place the changing mat or in a nappy stacker close by.

■ Keep a nappy and wipes out so they are always to hand.

If your baby is going to sleep in his own room, you could get a small put-up bed so one parent can sleep there if necessary.

Ways of spending less

A baby magazine recently calculated that parents spend at least £4,000 on their baby in his first year. And that's a conservative guess: it doesn't include the cost of childcare or any luxuries. Not everyone can afford to be blasé about such a sum.

If you can't beg, steal or borrow from friends, buying second hand is your best bet. You can pick up most things on the Internet or you could try your local edition of *Loot*, and there are bargains to be found at National Childbirth Trust (NCT) sales. Local twins-club sales are another little known and underrated source of baby equipment.

The bigger supermarkets usually stock a range of baby items at reasonable prices. There is stiff competition between online distributors selling baby equipment and there are bargains to be found if you have time to surf. You can also hire key equipment, which will also save you the hassle of finding storage space for things when they are no longer needed.

Last-minute things you could do before the birth (if this is your first baby and you have time on your hands)

■ Clean the house
■ Prepare as many meals as you can and freeze them
■ Stock up on local take-away or delivery menus

- Set up an Internet supermarket account if you haven't already done so
- Test out any baby equipment that looks complicated
- Practise getting the car seat and pushchair in and out of the car
- Get a hands-free phone with an answer machine to screen calls
- Get a tumble drier if you don't have one
- Talk to mums to pick up tips
- Browse parenting websites for information, advice and chatboards
- Think ahead about feeding and routines so you are clear about your choices
- Read up about a baby's first weeks/months of life
- Make a list of people you'll want to call from hospital
- Investigate local daycare providers (if you think you might need one)
- Prepare your hospital bag. Don't leave it too late . . .

Preparing your hospital bag

This list is a prompt to help you decide what you may need, but some items are a matter of personal choice.

- Coins for the hospital car park and phone
- List of phone numbers of people to ring
- Radio with headphones in case you can't sleep
- Ear plugs to shut out the hubbub of the ward
- Magazines or books
- Camera and film
- Bag of toiletries
- Make-up
- Hairbrush and hairdryer

- Small mirror
- Dressing gown, slippers, socks
- Old nightdress to wear in labour
- Nightdress, preferably something that unbuttons at the front
- Paper pants or Bridget Jones-style loose-fitting pants (particularly if you have a caesarean – they don't rub on the wound)
- Nursing bra
- Flip flops to use in the ward and in the shower or bathroom
- Toilet paper (if you crave little luxuries)
- Tissues
- Maternity pads (for post-delivery bleeding)
- Breast pads
- Nipple shields (in case your nipples get sore)
- Mints (in case you can't brush your teeth)
- Nappies as hospitals don't always supply them
- Baby clothes, including a going-home outfit
- Clothes you'll wear to go home
- Baby car seat

2.

Getting off to a Flying Start

'I can't be the only mother who has wondered, at some stage in the first few days after a baby arrives, "Why did no one tell me it would be like this?"

'I assumed someone would show me what to do: when to feed, when to bath, when to change a nappy, when to sleep . . . But they didn't. I felt foolish asking basic questions and got into a complete muddle. I was so clueless, in fact, that I thought new babies needed to be kept indoors with the curtains closed, so that's what I did with mine – for a week. No wonder they developed jaundice from a lack of daylight.

'If you have no idea what to do, you are not alone . . .

'That's where this chapter comes in. It will get you going, answer the questions you might not like to ask, and give you tips on making things run smoothly.

'We've avoided going into detail on the birth itself (there's plenty of information elsewhere), but we have some brief pre-birth and post-birth advice for mums and dads before moving on to babies and babycare.

'After that comes feeding in the first couple of weeks, including guidance on laying the foundations for a feeding routine. (You can move on to a routine any time after your baby has reached about two weeks; the next chapter will show you how.)

'Finally . . . advice on sleep. Jo has "secrets" to share on what you can do to get your baby working towards good sleeping patterns even at this early age (chapters 7–10 will show you what you can do to get your baby sleeping through the night).

'Even if you're not a first-time parent we hope and believe that you will find much of this advice refreshing and useful.'

Barbara

Before the birth

Opting for a home birth

Only about one in fifty births in the UK takes place at home, but many more women – about one in five it's thought – would consider a home birth if they felt more confident they would get the support they need.

A home birth may suit you if you have older children and are reluctant to leave them for a hospital stay; or you may feel that a home birth offers you the best chance of having a midwife present throughout your labour. Some mums choose this option in the hope that it increases the likelihood of having a vaginal delivery without an epidural. For many though it is simply that the comforts and benefits of being at home are preferable to the clinical environment of a hospital and the hubbub of a busy labour ward.

Whatever your reasons, you are entitled to have a home birth. But an entitlement to a home birth doesn't always mean that getting one is easy: unfortunately, resistance is still to be found throughout the health service. A shortage of midwives is sometimes cited as a factor for refusing a home birth (it is usual, but not obligatory, to have two midwives present, although there is no evidence that it improves the outcome), but don't be put off if your first enquiry is not greeted with enthusiasm.

Your GP's agreement for a home birth is not a requirement and, if you find his or her support lacking, it might be best to approach your community midwife or community midwifery manager directly. (All maternity units have to provide a home-birth service.) In fact you don't need to involve your GP in your maternity care at all if you don't want to, in which case you could make your community midwife your first port of call. You could also try the NCT for advice – many local branches have home-birth support groups and will know who is likely to be helpful locally – or contact AIMS, the Association for Improvements in the Maternity Services.

Women opting for a home birth through the NHS are usually looked after by a small team of community midwives so there is some continuity of care. A midwife from the team will be assigned to you, but there is no guarantee that she will be with you at the birth. One option to ease the way for a home birth and to guarantee absolutely that you will know the midwife who will be present at the birth is to hire an independent midwife, although this doesn't come cheap and will cost upwards of £2,000. The fee covers all pre-birth consultations and twenty-eight days of follow-up appointments. If complications arise during the birth and you need to go to hospital she will stay with you throughout, working alongside the hospital medical team in a supportive role and as an advocate for you.

Midwives bring everything needed for the birth and clear up afterwards (including taking away the placenta unless you want to keep it), but it's up to you to arrange for a birthing pool if you want one. There are companies which hire these out.

Remember that if you give birth at home your partner and family aren't restricted by hospital visiting hours, but nor are other visitors who might drop by unannounced just when you're trying to rest. You could put a bunch of balloons on your door to announce the new arrival, along with a note suggesting times when visitors are welcome.

Opting for an independent midwife or doula

The lack of continuity of care for hospital births may explain why some women choose to pay to have a professional by their side at the birth. An independent midwife can see you through your pregnancy and work alongside a hospital team during the birth. But that luxury comes at a price (see above).

A less expensive option is a birth doula. Birth doulas are not medically qualified but are experienced in looking after both mum and dad before, during and after the birth. The doula can explain what your options are and help you draw up a birth plan, then act as your 'spokesman' to the medical team during labour, reminding them of your preferences. She will usually be available to you for a short time after the birth, helping with breastfeeding and visiting you once you are home.

Dads and the birth

'What did I do to help my wife at the birth?
'I agreed with everything she said and did everything she asked me to.'
Tom

The birth of a baby is incredibly exciting, but can also be traumatic and exhausting – for dads as well as mums. Dads are suddenly faced with caring for two very needy people and often feel as if they are shouldering all the responsibility.

Here are a few ideas of things dads can do to make things run more smoothly.

- Check the route to the hospital before the birth so you know how long it takes to get there (and you don't get lost)
- Stock the freezer with food
- Pre-pack a bag with magazines, snacks, drinks, cards, camera, small change for phones/vending machines
- Keep your pager or mobile battery well-charged
- Prepare a list of the phone numbers you'll want to ring.

Not to mention doing a bit of homework on the birthing process: you may feel better for being informed, and your partner may feel better if you know what you're talking about. If decisions need to be made, you may have to take charge and if your partner is not getting what she wants you may have to insist that she gets it. How you do your homework is up to you. Here are two different views:

> 'I didn't relish the idea of going on an antenatal course, but I'm really glad I did. It meant that during the birth I knew what we could ask for and what we could refuse. When my wife was offered an epidural I felt I knew enough to say no. In the end she did have one, but by then we were happy with the decision.'
> **Roger**

> 'We'd been to antenatal classes, but all they did was lull us into a false sense of security. There was a huge gap between the fantasy world they conjured up and the reality of an overstretched maternity ward. When things started to go wrong during Jane's labour, I had to fight to find someone who really knew what they were doing. What we'd learned at the classes turned out to be useless.'
> **Richard**

Childbirth can be a strange experience for dads, producing reactions ranging from joy to terror, apathy to a sense of isolation. Whether you are feeling tired, worried or angry, you need to let your partner know that you are calm, you are on her side and that you think she is doing a brilliant job. This is not as easy as it sounds, especially if you have to endure (at second hand) hours of painful and exhausting labour.

Although this is a time when the little things you do can make a difference, it may also be a time when mothers forget to say thank you. That's the fate of the supporting cast: they hardly ever get the bouquets. But there's no reason why that should make the experience any less exciting.

> *'I tried to keep in my head that I should be thinking of Kate — but that went out the window the moment I saw the baby. I felt like a champagne bottle popping open with all my emotions shooting through the top. It was so overwhelming that I cried . . .'*
> **Tom**

Try to take responsibility for keeping visitors in order, and accept that you may feel left out of the action as they coo over the baby, congratulate the mother and ignore the chap in the corner. Grit your teeth and enjoy the reflected glory.

Don't rely on the hospital taking a share of the load. Few hospitals can devote as much time to healthy mothers and babies as dads might like, and that leaves them (literally, sometimes) holding the baby, changing the baby or even bathing the baby to give mum a break. Midwives come and go in a most disconcerting way, and it may fall to you again to make sure that your partner gets what she needs — a cup of tea, a new packet of tissues, or some help with breastfeeding.

Finally, do make sure that the house is clean and tidy before your partner comes home. It matters to mums more than most dads realize.

After the birth

Your body

If you have had stitches after a vaginal delivery you may feel quite uncomfortable. Some women find that the discomfort in the first few days is alleviated by sitting on a rubber swim ring. Urinating can be difficult: try pouring a jug of warm water over your stitches while you are on the loo to ease the pain, or urinate in the bath. You could add some rock salt to the water to act as an antiseptic and use a hairdryer on your stitches afterwards to make sure they are really dry. Try holding a pack of frozen peas (wrapped in a towel) on your stitches for a couple of minutes. Remove it, then repeat a couple of times.

Don't make the assumption that a vaginal delivery is always easier to get over than a caesarean; in some cases it isn't.

'With my first child I had a vaginal delivery. I was in labour for sixteen hours, pushing for six of them, and with only gas-and-air for pain relief. It took a long time to get over the physical and emotional trauma of the birth. I was very uncomfortable down below and couldn't sit properly for about six weeks.

'With my second child it was very different. After about an hour of labour I needed an emergency caesarean. The whole process was very calm, and I even managed to catch a glimpse of my daughter being born, something I had missed out on with my son. The operation itself was much easier to recover from. Although my tummy was a bit uncomfortable, after three weeks I was back to normal and

able to drive. I was amazed, especially given the negative press that caesareans get.'
Lucie

If you've had an emergency caesarean preceded by a long labour you will be exhausted, and you may also be disappointed that you didn't deliver your baby vaginally. If the birth was traumatic, you could be in a state of shock too. To ease your mind it sometimes helps to talk through what happened with a midwife or obstetrician and find out why it was necessary.

Once the anaesthetic wears off, a caesarean – whether emergency or elective – can leave you sore and restricted in your movements. Coughing or laughing (and pooing) can be agonizing – hold your wound when you do so to ease the pressure on it. Your Bridget Jones-style knickers will now come into their own: anything smaller may rub the stitches.

Some women though are up on their feet within hours and report little discomfort, so take heart and hope that you may be one of them. Hospital staff will make you get up within hours of the operation however you feel in order to speed your recovery and help your circulation. You will be given support tights to prevent blood clots. Yes, they are hideous, but keep them on until advised that you can remove them. You will probably be kept in hospital for longer than you had planned – delaying your longed-for return home. If you lost a lot of blood during the operation and your blood count is low you will feel truly dreadful. Your option will be iron supplements or, in more severe cases, a blood transfusion.

As if all that were not enough to dampen what should be joyous spirits, the sight of your wound can be a shock. Some women swear by arnica tablets (a homeopathic remedy) to speed up the healing process. You should take them just before the operation if you can, and for at least a week afterwards. You can also get arnica oil or horse chestnut oil for your bath. Applying pure vitamin E oil to the wound as soon as possible helps soften scar tissue as it forms. Your scar will, over time, diminish and fade.

Try not to lose sight of the fact that you have had major surgery and that you need to rest as much as possible, especially in the first two weeks (and probably a bit beyond). You can help yourself by lying flat for a spell every day to take the pressure off your wound.

Don't lift *anything* except your baby and under no circumstances push a pram until you are ready. Wounds sometimes reopen. If you find your wound is weeping or gaping, speak to your midwife or doctor. Don't drive until you feel ready (you may find it hard to brake in an emergency). It is not illegal to drive after a caesarean but if you have an accident and it is shown that you were not fit you can run into trouble with your insurance. Avoid any exercise until at least six weeks after the birth and your postnatal check-up.

It can take months to feel completely back to normal after a caesarean, but the intense discomfort of the first few days disappears rapidly.

Your feelings

Many new mums become tearful a few days after the birth, which is not surprising considering the stress of childbirth and the heightened emotions that overwhelm you once you hold your new baby in your arms. Add to that a few sleepless nights and it is a heady mix. It is thought that more than 80 per cent of mothers get the 'baby blues'.

The baby blues usually pass after a couple of weeks, although any new mum will probably continue to have some tearful moments in the first few months of her baby's life. Life with a newborn baby is a struggle at times: it can be isolating, frustrating and exhausting, and if this is your first baby it may take you many months to adjust to the idea of being a parent. However strong your love for your baby, you may be resentful at times at the way your life has changed and at the loss of your freedom and independence. It is sometimes hard to share these concerns even with your partner and a new mum can think she is the only mother who feels this way. Try to meet and talk to other mothers with small babies as soon as you can get out and about. Your midwife or health visitor will know of local mother-and-baby groups.

If you find the baby blues linger longer than a couple of weeks you might be at risk of postnatal depression. Don't ignore how you feel – there is advice on p. 212.

You may also be anxious, particularly if this is your first baby, aware as you are of the massive responsibility you are now shouldering for this tiny human life. Or you may feel elated and on a permanent 'high'. Whatever your emotions, they will be intense, and whatever you may have been led to believe, bonding with a baby isn't always instantaneous. It will come in time, but if you find it doesn't happen as soon as you had expected, don't worry.

'In the first few days after the birth I felt elated and terrified at the same time. I started to have nightmares about my babies dying through my incompetence. The fear of losing them was overwhelming and I would start crying, only minutes after I had been on a complete high. I have never experienced anything like it. It was a wonderful but very anxious time.'
Barbara

Baby basics

Nappy know-how

A newborn baby's nappy should be changed around seven or eight times every twenty-four hours and after every poo. Change your baby before his feed as this will wake him up and make him more comfortable while feeding. If your baby is screaming before his feed, you could wait to change him – maybe halfway through a feed or between breasts, if you are breastfeeding – which has the added advantage of keeping him awake for the whole feed.

Your baby's skin needs to be wiped at each change even if it's not very wet. Urine is acidic and can irritate the skin. In the first couple of weeks, use cotton wool and water rather than baby wipes for nappy changes – a newborn baby's skin is very sensitive. Use cotton wool or a towel to dry the skin afterwards. Some parents prefer to continue with cotton wool and water for several months. After a poo, use an antiseptic barrier cream or soothing cream if there is any sign of irritation.

As your baby gets older and the number of his daily feeds decreases you can reduce the number of nappy changes accordingly to coincide with the feeds.

Bathing your baby

The first time you bath a baby it may feel strange: holding a slippery, naked baby can be unnerving and it may take a while before you feel confident and comfortable about bathtime. You can top 'n' tail your baby for the first couple of weeks if you prefer (see below).

Bathtime is a key part of a baby's bedtime ritual (see p. 94) so is best done at night. Bathing your baby at the same time every day becomes a cue that bedtime and sleep time are approaching. As your baby grows, it will also provide an opportunity for him to let off steam and exercise his legs by kicking and splashing.

You can use a baby bath at the beginning: either place it on the floor or get one that props on top of your bath. Babies outgrow baby baths by the age of about three months. Alternatively, move straight to a baby bath seat placed inside your own bath.

You will also need:

- Cotton wool
- Warm water
- Two towels (one for the baby to lie on and one to wrap him in)
- A clean nappy
- Clean clothes
- Aqueous cream to moisturize his skin
- Aqueous cream, baby massage oil or grapeseed oil if you want to massage him (see below).

To bath your baby:

- Lay him on a towel (or changing mat) on the floor or on a safe surface.
- Strip him down to his nappy.
- Wrap him in the other towel as if swaddling him.
- Using damp cotton wool wipe his eyes, from the inner side of the eye outwards towards the ear. Use a fresh piece of cotton wool for each eye.
- Wipe your baby's face and under his chin (where milk deposits can gather).
- Use small circular strokes on his head; this can help to prevent cradle cap (see p. 202).

- Take off his nappy and wipe his bottom.
- Put him in the bath, having checked the water temperature with your elbow (it should feel warm) or preferably with a thermometer (it should be no higher than 97°F). The water should be no deeper than about 4 in.
- Trickle water over him gently using your hands or a sponge. As your baby grows you can start to use a sponge to wipe him, and introduce toys to bathtime.
- Pour water over his hair.
- Take your baby out of the bath.
- Wrap him in a towel and lay him on the towel or changing mat you used before.
- Dry him and put on his nappy.
- Turn him on to his tummy and take away the wet towel.
- Dry his hair and moisturize his skin.
- Give him a massage once he is over about four weeks.
- Dress him.

You don't need to use baby bath products on a newborn baby; they may dry the skin or cause irritation. If you feel the need to add something to the water make sure the products are unscented and hypoallergenic, or try some Oilatum oil. Save other products until your baby is three months old and always check that no irritation occurs.

Top 'n' tailing your baby

You don't need to bath your new baby every day; every two to three days is fine. For the first few weeks you could just top 'n' tail him in the evenings. You should also top 'n' tail your baby every morning until he is around six months old.

You will need:

- Cotton wool
- Warm water
- Two towels (one for the baby to lie on and one to wrap him in)
- A clean nappy
- Clean clothes
- Aqueous cream to moisturize his skin
- Aqueous cream, baby massage oil or grapeseed oil if you want to massage him (see below).

To top 'n' tail your baby:
- Lay him on the towel (or changing mat) on the floor or on a safe surface.
- Strip him down to his vest and nappy (if you are going to massage him, take his vest off too).
- Wrap him in the towel as if swaddling him.
- Using damp cotton wool wipe both eyes, from the inner side of the eye outwards towards the ear. Use a fresh piece of cotton wool for each eye.
- Wipe your baby's face and under his chin (where milk deposits can gather).
- Use small circular strokes on his head; this can help to prevent cradle cap (see p. 202).
- Wipe him dry with the towel.
- Take off his nappy and wipe his bottom, paying particular attention to the creases.
- Dry and moisturize the skin and put on a new nappy.
- Massage your baby (night-time) once he is over about four weeks.
- Dress him.

Baby massage

Once your baby is about four weeks old you can introduce him to a massage.

Baby massage is becoming very popular and there are books on it and courses you can attend to learn about different massage strokes and their benefits. Your midwife or health visitor should know about local baby massage classes and may even have a leaflet to guide you while you get started. Research suggests that massage is calming for babies and good for their health; it also helps bonding and may even reduce postnatal depression.

Massaging a baby does not need to be complicated. Here is a quick, easy and straightforward method. Lay your baby on his back on his changing mat or on a towel on a safe surface, preferably with his feet closest to you, head furthest away, and with good eye contact. You will need some aqueous cream, baby massage oil or grapeseed oil. Using both your hands stroke each leg from thigh to toes for about a minute, and then each arm from shoulder to fingers for another minute, with firm, smooth, squeezing movements. Then massage his tummy in a clockwise motion to help alleviate tummy ache and wind (this replicates the direction of the intestine where the wind collects). Turn him on to his tummy and rub his back gently from the bottom up to his neck for another minute. This position has the added benefit of strengthening his neck muscles. You can then turn him over and massage his feet and toes gently.

Mums usually love baby massage too, although it may not be everyone's cup of tea. Sometimes it doesn't appeal to babies either. If yours reacts by crying (which some do), wait a few days and try again. It is worth persevering because babies usually learn to love it and it can become one of the best parts of their day.

Dressing your baby

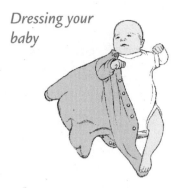

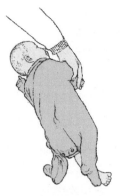

1. Lay your baby on his mat and put one arm and one leg into the babygro on the side nearest you

2. Now roll your baby away from you on to his side while tucking the babygro halfway underneath him

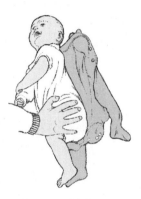

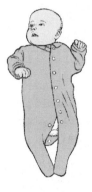

3. Roll him back towards you on to his other side while you pull the babygro out from underneath him and he is now lying on it

4. Put the other arm and leg in and fasten poppers

None of us likes to feel we have to be shown how to carry out the simplest tasks, but it's worth learning the trick of putting on a babygro. This really is the easiest way to do it, especially with a wriggling baby. Lay your baby on his mat and put one arm and one leg into the babygro on the side nearest to you. Now roll your baby away from you on to his side while tucking the babygro halfway underneath him. Roll him back towards you on to his other side while you pull the babygro out from underneath him and he is now lying on it. Put the other arm and leg in and fasten the poppers.

Dummies/Soothers

Many parents hate dummies because they think they are dirty, a sign of lazy parenting or a habit that can never be dropped and so is best avoided altogether. But dummies can be a godsend, particularly with a 'sucky' or unsettled baby, or with multiples, and they need not become a habit if you use them at the right time of day or night and remove them when your baby is around four months old (adjust for prematurity). This is when a baby's sucking reflex disappears – and with it his need for a dummy.

'I suggest to parents that they restrict dummies to the following situations:

- During the day when a baby simply can't settle for a nap (but use as a last, rather than as a first, resort)
- During the day if your baby is very irritable before a feed
- At night when a baby can't be soothed by other methods (but use as a last, rather than as a first, resort)
- At night to help stretch a baby's feeds (see chapter 9) with a view to getting him to sleep through the night
- to relieve a baby who has bad wind and in particular a baby who has colic.

Sucking seems to ease a baby's tummy pains.

'When babies reach about four months I suggest withdrawing the dummy during the day for a few days

before withdrawing it at night. It usually takes only a couple of nights of being unsettled before a baby forgets he ever had one. If you do this now, you will save yourself much trauma later.'
Jo

It is very important not to let your baby get into the habit of using his dummy to help him to fall asleep, otherwise he will come to rely on it and be unable to fall asleep without it. He needs to learn always to fall asleep by himself, which is why a dummy should be used to help settle a baby as a last, rather than a first, resort.

Always sterilize dummies. Some brands have plastic tops to keep the dummy clean. Never put them in your own mouth (it is full of bacteria, which your baby may not appreciate) or wash them under the tap, and never put anything on them (parents are known to coat them in honey or something sweet).

Tummy time

Although it is strongly recommended that babies sleep on their backs as this reduces the risk of cot death, babies need to spend some time on their tummies in order to strengthen their neck and back muscles. (Even a short tummy time every day can also help to alleviate the problem of head flattening that happens when babies spend a lot of time on their backs.)

From the age of about four weeks place your baby on his tummy on a blanket on the floor during his play time. He may protest at first: it will feel strange to him and he will have to work extra hard to hold his head up, but he will get used to it. Start with a few minutes a day and build to about thirty minutes by the age of four to six months. Keep doing this until your baby can crawl.

A good time of day to opt for tummy time is the late afternoon. A baby – especially in the first couple of months – can get tummy ache from wind at this time of day and be very grizzly. The pressure of lying on his tummy can bring relief.

Never leave him unattended and don't let him fall asleep.

Feeding

Signs of hunger in babies

- Rooting – turning his head towards your (or anyone's) breast (*newborns only*)
- Head butting your (or anyone's) shoulder (*newborns only*)
- Grabbing on to your finger if you place it in his mouth (*newborns only*)
- Pushing his fists or fingers into his mouth (this happens both when babies are hungry and when they are tired because they come to associate feeding with sleeping, so look for other signs of hunger too)
- Restlessness
- Grunting
- Sucking briefly if you place a dummy in his mouth, then shaking his head from side to side in frustration
- Opening his mouth wide and crying
- Short sharp cries on and off
- Sucking on any clothing that is within reach.

As your baby grows you will start to identify his hunger cues quickly and easily.

Breastfeeding: getting going

'The birth of my twins (one of whom fed readily at the breast while the other refused), taught me two important lessons: first, breastfeeding doesn't come easily to every mother and baby, and second, when there is a problem there isn't always a sympathetic or knowledgeable voice to turn to. My pleas (to the midwives) for help were met with little interest, which made me feel I should be able to sort things out myself or admit to defeat. It took time but I found a way through: if I hadn't I would have had to live with regret. I went on to breastfeed successfully for several months and absolutely loved it.

'I have since spoken to dozens of mums and discovered that my experience was not unique. Some mums do struggle with something they had always assumed would come easily; and they are taken aback when it doesn't. If this happens, you may find that health professionals – to whom you will automatically turn – offer you inexpert and conflicting advice. This can leave you distressed and anxious and at risk of giving up altogether, while your baby gets hungry and frustrated. Which is very sad because expert, specialist breastfeeding guidance can usually resolve problems very quickly. But that advice can prove elusive.

'If you and your baby take to breastfeeding readily, it is of course a joy. But if you don't, please ask for, or demand, the help you need. There are some ideas in this section on where to look and some stories to show neither you nor I are alone.'

Barbara

'When I struggled with breastfeeding the midwife's casual response was, "You've got the wrong type of nipple". I burst into tears.'
Hannah

'The biggest mistake I made was leaving hospital before the breastfeeding was properly established. They told me it would "work out" but it didn't and whenever I rang them from home they couldn't really help me. I ended up in tears at one point not knowing what to do. Luckily I did sort it in the end, but after much heartache.'
Rebecca

It takes two to breastfeed. Which means both of you will suffer if it doesn't click immediately. A baby who cannot latch on to the breast gets frustrated, miserable and thirsty, which in turn is very upsetting for a mother. Very few health professionals (including midwives) receive specialist training in breastfeeding and it *is* an area that requires expertise. Some hospitals have breastfeeding counsellors with the knowledge needed – but they may not be available at the moment you need them. Once you're home you should find a local drop-in clinic with a trained adviser – and with luck it will have baby-friendly opening hours. Hospitals which boast accreditation by the Unicef Baby Friendly Initiative usually have helpful policies regarding breastfeeding support. Your maternity unit will be able to provide you with information about all these services. Getting your breastfeeding established early is important so don't delay in seeking help if you need to.

If your hospital services are lacking, you could contact a telephone support line where you can talk to a trained counsellor. If you still can't get what you need, one option is to pay for a private lactation specialist to visit you at home. They are thin on the ground but the Lactation Consultants of Great Britain should be able to help find you one. If breastfeeding really matters to you and you are struggling, it may be a small price to pay (see Notes, p. 288, for further information).

'When Franklin was born I couldn't get him to latch on but I got no help at the hospital. The midwives all had different techniques and tips. The advice I got from one was: "When he's ready to drink he'll do it." Which he didn't. It was very laissez-faire. It was hot on the ward and Franklin was parched. He cried every time he came near my breast but couldn't drink. Nobody told me what to do. They didn't want to give him a bottle because they didn't want to be responsible for doing so, yet there were no suggestions for doing anything else.

'He began to lose weight and I was completely distraught. When he was ten days old I had all but given up – so we called a private lactation expert. Within fifteen minutes of her being with us Franklin was breastfeeding. It was really amazing. She showed me how milk flowed from the breast and how to get the baby's mouth around the nipple. She explained that this is a very specialized area – getting a midwife to show you what to do would be like getting a GP to do an eye operation!

'Confidence is the key. We had no "technical" problems: we just needed to be shown what to do. If someone had come into my room at the hospital after Franklin was born he would have been breastfeeding straight away. It cost me £90 and was worth every penny.'
Josephine

If you find breastfeeding tricky at first, remember that it does get easier as time goes by: the first ten days are usually the hardest.

Sore nipples should disappear after this time. Then you can start really enjoying to feed your baby. Sadly many mums give up in the first week. If you find it hard, don't give up too quickly; try to persevere for at least ten days before deciding.

None of this is meant to suggest that you *will* encounter problems; chances are that you won't and you will go on to breastfeed your baby successfully for many months.

How often do I breastfeed my baby in the first two weeks?

A newborn baby needs to be fed little and often. If you are breastfeeding this will also build up your milk supply. Newborns are very sleepy though, and can sleep for long stretches of up to five hours at a time. Mothers often assume they need to feed their baby only when he wakes, but this is not advisable. Not only will your baby not be taking the food he needs, but your breasts will not be getting the stimulation they need to get your milk supply established. When your baby stops being so sleepy at about two weeks, he may find there is not enough milk to satisfy his hunger. Babies who are born before term are often particularly sleepy but still need regular feeding, and if they are in special care you will need an expressing machine to supply your own milk. (Hand expressing your colostrum is advised until your milk comes in; this has also been shown to help achieve successful breastfeeding.)

Midwives usually advise mothers to keep their baby on the breast for as long as he wants, which can spell disaster. Some babies are particularly 'sucky' and will stay on the breast long after they have taken the milk they need. These babies may cry when taken off, leading their mums to put them back on, believing that they are still hungry. The babies drink/suck on and off for hours, which exhausts them. A newborn baby cannot stay awake for more than one to one-and-a-half hours without getting overtired, and overtired babies cannot sleep. Their mothers get exhausted too and the constant feeding makes their nipples sore and very painful.

> '*I had no problems getting my baby latched on. But no one prepared me for my particular predicament, which was that Leo either seemed to take great comfort in sucking on me for hours, or he was a very hungry baby and was never satisfied after feeding on me. I remember asking the midwives how long it was reasonable for a baby to be nursing, and never seemed to get a clear answer. You were made to feel you just had to nurse until your baby came off looking satisfied, or if it took comfort in sucking on you, let it! At times he would be on the breast for up to four hours . . .*'
> **Mandy**

> '*When Lydia was born they told me to keep her on the breast for as long as she wanted but sometimes she would still be there an hour and a half later. My nipples were so sore I was tempted to give up breastfeeding altogether. I didn't realize that she wasn't actually feeding the whole time – she was just sucking for comfort.*'
> **Annabel**

If this happens, you need to work out when your baby has stopped drinking and is sucking for comfort (see below). Equally, you need to be aware that if your baby seems to want feeding very frequently, there may be other reasons for his crying: he could be very tired – perhaps from sucking so much.

Jo's breastfeeding guidance for weeks 1 and 2

Your milk usually comes in on day 3 or 4. Before that your baby will be getting colostrum, which is rich in antibodies. If you have had a caesarean your milk may come in a little later. Most women know immediately: their breasts become very full and hard. If they are very painful, express a little off each side before feeding. If you are not sure, try expressing to see if you are producing milk. You should notice your baby following a pattern of sucking and swallowing once he is drinking milk.

Days 1 and 2

Ideally your baby should be put to the breast very soon after he is born (assuming he is not premature and has to go into special care).

Give him around five minutes on each breast every time he is hungry. He may be sleeping a lot during this time, but try not to let him go for more than three hours without a feed.

Don't express during this time.

Days 3 and 4

Give your baby around ten minutes on one breast and five minutes on the other every time he is hungry. This will probably be about every two hours. Don't let your baby go any longer than three hours or he won't be drinking enough. You may have to wake him to feed.

Once your milk has come in you could express from both breasts after each feed to help build up your supply. Don't worry if the amounts are small at first. Store the milk in a freezer, but use it soon – at most within a week. This early milk will still have some colostrum in it and should be given to a baby in the first few days of life. For example, use it to top your baby up in the early evening when mums' milk supply is often at its lowest.

If your milk hasn't come in, keep feeding as above until it does, but don't start to express until it has.

Babies sometimes get hungry while waiting for mum's milk to come in. You may be advised to give him formula; don't feel this means the end of your breastfeeding. Keep putting your baby to the breast when he is hungry before offering a bottle.

Jaundiced babies or babies with low blood sugar levels may also be given formula on medical advice. Again, don't assume this means that breastfeeding is no longer possible.

Days 5–7

Give your baby fifteen minutes on one side and let him take the second breast if he seems to want more milk. Do this every time he is hungry but try to work towards not doing it more frequently than every two and a half hours. A healthy baby born at a good weight should be able to last two and a half hours after a full feed. Feeding more frequently will exhaust him.

Don't let your baby go any longer than three hours between feeds during the day or he won't be drinking enough. You may have to wake him. He may go longer in between feeds at night if he has drunk well during the day. This is fine, but if he is under 6lb he should be woken to feed every three hours at night too.

Express on both sides after he has finished, until both breasts are empty.

Days 8–14

Your milk should be flowing now and your baby can probably get enough milk in the first thirty to forty-five minutes if he is sucking consistently. But bear in mind that all babies are different; you will soon work out how long your baby needs to take a full feed.

Feed your baby every two and a half to three hours. Babies who take a full feed should be able to go for that long in between feeds. Try not to let your baby feed more frequently or a pattern of snacking will set in.

Don't let your baby go any longer than three hours during the day without feeding or he won't be drinking enough. He may go longer in between feeds at night if he has drunk well during the day. This is fine, but if he is under 6lb he should be woken to feed every three hours at night too.

Start to take a note now of the times in between feeds, as well as of your baby's sleeping patterns, to give you some guidance on which routine to follow. (Don't be surprised, though, if your baby doesn't follow a pattern that is easy to recognize, particularly a feeding pattern. Some babies don't, and need to be guided into a feeding routine.)

Once your breastfeeding is established, which should be after about ten days, you can start thinking about feeding your baby on a routine (see chapter 4). At around two weeks (and if he is over 7lb) you can also start to follow the advice in chapter 9 on stretching your baby's night-time feeds and working towards a night of unbroken sleep.

Should I express my milk?

In some cases expressing can help enormously. When your milk comes in, your breasts may be very full and painful, and expressing an ounce off each side before each feed will ease the discomfort. (Don't express before your milk comes in.)

Expressing is useful when you have a sleepy baby who isn't too hungry in the first couple of weeks and who doesn't drink much at each feed. This may mean your breasts won't be stimulated enough just at the point where you are trying to get your milk supply going. When your baby stops being so sleepy he may find there isn't enough milk to satisfy his hunger. It's at this point that mums often assume they don't have enough milk for their baby and give up breastfeeding altogether. Expressing after each feed in the early days can help to get round this.

Once your breastfeeding is established, you can continue to express. Many mums find that the best time to do this is early in the morning when their breasts are very full or just before going to bed (especially if you opt to give this as a formula feed – see page 155). You may find your expressed milk particularly useful when you give your baby his 7 p.m. feed before he goes to bed. A lot of mums find their milk supply is low at this time of day.

Breast milk will keep twenty-four hours in a fridge and can be frozen for up to three months. Thawed milk can be kept in the fridge for up to twelve hours.

How do I know when my baby has taken a full feed?

Getting your baby to take a full feed every time is really important if you are to establish a routine and regular feeding patterns. Otherwise the habit of snacking will set in, and with it will come irregular sleep patterns, a tired baby and a tired you.

Every baby is different, so you will need to work out his pattern. Check if he is sucking and swallowing consistently. If he isn't, you need to take him off and latch him on again. You also need to be sure that he is fully awake. Check that his last feed was at least two and a half hours before – otherwise he won't be hungry and won't suck at each feed consistently. He needs to drain one breast, so he takes both the foremilk (which is watery and thirst-quenching) and the creamy hindmilk (which satisfies his hunger and helps him to gain weight). Don't be surprised if, in the first couple of weeks, your baby takes up to forty-five minutes to feed.

Most babies take a full feed from one breast in the first three to four weeks, although you can always offer the second breast if your baby still seems hungry. After that age they usually need to be offered the second breast at every feed.

Your breast will feel soft to the touch when it has been drained. If you are not sure whether your baby has finished feeding, it is advisable to limit feeds in the first six weeks to about an hour and after that to forty-five minutes. If your baby screams when he is taken off the breast after that he is probably not hungry, but tired from all the sucking. Try giving him a dummy to calm him. Once he is calm, take it away so he doesn't use it to help himself fall asleep.

How do I keep a sleepy baby awake for a breastfeed?

New babies (and in particular premature or low-birthweight babies) are very sleepy for a couple of weeks and may doze off after a few minutes of feeding. They need to be woken up to keep drinking or they won't take a full feed and will be hungry again soon after. If your baby gets into the habit of falling asleep on the breast, there's a risk he will start to associate feeding with falling asleep which is not a good association; he may learn he can fall asleep only if he has your breast to suck on. Wake him up and lay him down to sleep still awake.

Try these techniques to keep a baby awake for a feed:

- Change his nappy before feeding. This has the added benefit that he will be clean and dry for his meal
- Tickle your baby under his chin
- Take your baby's foot out of his babygro and tickle it
- Blow gently on his face
- Lay him on his changing mat or next to you on the sofa.

What if my baby won't latch on?

The rugby-tackle breastfeeding hold (holding your baby's legs under your arm) can make it easier for your baby to latch on. If he doesn't, take him off and try again. It may take several attempts to succeed.

Babies can find it difficult to latch on to very full breasts. You can either express a small amount before the feed or you can put a warm flannel on the breast immediately before your baby feeds to make the milk flow more quickly and reduce your baby's workload.

For small and premature babies in particular, latching on and sucking are hard work.

'I know from experience that having a baby who refuses to – or can't – latch on is very upsetting. When this happened with one of my twins (who was very small at birth) and when advice at the hospital was not forthcoming, a friend suggested expressing my milk and giving it to him in a bottle. I set myself a limit to how long I would try my baby on the breast – fifteen minutes – and then I would offer him the bottle of expressed milk. This reduced my stress levels because I knew he was getting my milk, which was the key thing. And it meant that my milk kept flowing, which in the long run was a boon.

'It took about four weeks before he latched on – after that he took either breast or bottle very happily.'
Barbara

Nipple/teat confusion

Mothers are often advised not to give their new baby a bottle in case it causes him subsequently to reject the nipple (breastfeeding requires more work on a baby's part than a bottle). So if you have a small baby who finds it hard to latch on to the breast, or if you are medically required to feed him formula before your milk comes in, you may be advised to feed from a cup.

It can be disheartening to see a small baby sitting on your knee having milk poured into his mouth. Besides, nipple/teat confusion is not always a risk. In fact, the opposite is more common: a baby who is never given a bottle (whether it be expressed milk or formula) in the early weeks of life can subsequently refuse bottles altogether. This can be quite stressful when it happens.

One way to avoid this problem is to give your baby a bottle once a day (either of expressed breastmilk or formula) once he reaches one or two weeks and once your breastfeeding is established. Try latex teats if he doesn't take to silicone teats. He will probably learn to love both the breast and the bottle.

Whenever a breastfed baby is given a bottle, and especially if this is in the first two weeks, don't be tempted to push it in his mouth, if his mouth doesn't open for it. Rub the teat along his lips (in the same way a breastfeeding baby can be teased with a nipple) and put the teat in once he opens his mouth. This will teach him that he has to 'work' for his milk (as he has to when he breastfeeds) and will stop him getting lazy on the breast. Most babies who get nipple/teat confusion have never been made to open their mouth wide to suck and so cannot latch on to a breast.

Breastfeeding tips

A quick guide to how to hold your baby to the breast is:

- Skin to chin – your skin should be touching the baby's chin
- Nipple to nose – your nipple should be just under his nose
- Tummy to mummy – his tummy should be across your tummy (unless you are doing the 'rugby tackle' hold).

Put baby to breast: never take your breast to the baby.

There are different types of breastfeeding holds you can try out to see which suits you and your baby best:

- The 'rugby tackle' hold, in which your baby's legs are under your arm
- The cradle hold: your baby is cradled in your arms across your body
- Lying down (helpful if you have had a caesarean).

A last word on breastfeeding: if you want to breastfeed and have made it clear that you do, your baby should not be given formula, even on medical advice, without your consent. If you are advised to give formula, make sure you understand and are happy with the advice before accepting it. Some hospitals require mums to sign a consent form before they will allow a baby to be given formula.

Foods to avoid when breastfeeding

Sometimes mums find that if they are breastfeeding and they eat certain foods, it can upset their baby a little. The most common culprits are:

- Garlic and onions (can give a baby colic-like symptoms)
- Strawberries (can cause a baby to get tummy ache)
- Dairy products. You may need to cut down on your dairy intake if your baby is showing signs of a dairy intolerance. Symptoms can include being sick a lot and developing eczema. (If these symptoms persist, seek medical advice to rule out reflux)
- Caffeine. Cut down or cut out, and in particular don't have caffeine after 5 p.m. – otherwise you may find you have a very wakeful baby
- Fizzy drinks, including champagne (although you may decide to avoid alcohol altogether). Don't have more than half a glass as it can give a baby tummy ache, and even cause him to be sick.

Bottle-feeding

If you are bottle-feeding, you can make up formula in advance to save time (it keeps for twenty-four hours in the fridge and you could make a whole jugful). Once you have warmed it, use it within an hour or discard it.

If you start bottle-feeding from the beginning you will need newborn teats, which have a slow flow speed; these are designed to let milk in at the speed at which a newborn baby can cope with it entering his mouth. As he gets stronger and more used to sucking, you can move up to a faster speed. If your baby is struggling to suck, you might find that latex, rather than silicone, teats will help.

Try to wash and sterilize bottles in the morning so you don't have a bottle crisis in the middle of the night.

For the first two weeks your baby will need to be fed little and often. This will be around every two and a half to three hours and he will need about 3 oz. Start to take a note of his feeding and sleeping patterns as soon as you can; this will help you to decide which routine to follow. You can start a bottle-fed baby on a routine when he is one to two weeks old (see chapter 4).

As with breastfeeding, it is really important that a baby takes his full bottle-feed at every feed or he will be hungry soon after and a pattern of snacking will set in along with all the accompanying disadvantages of feeding on demand.

How do I keep a sleepy baby awake for a bottle-feed?

New babies (and in particular premature or low-birthweight babies) are very sleepy for a couple of weeks and may doze off after a few minutes of feeding. They need to be woken up to keep drinking or they won't take a full feed and will be hungry again soon after. If your baby gets into the habit of falling asleep while on the bottle, there's a risk he will start to associate feeding with falling asleep which is not a good association; he may learn he can fall asleep only if he has a bottle for comfort. Wake him up and lay him down to sleep still awake.

Try these techniques to keep a baby awake for a feed:

- Wake your baby by changing his nappy before feeding. This has the added benefit that he will be clean and dry for his meal
- Tickle your baby under his chin
- Take your baby's foot out of his babygro and tickle it
- Blow gently on his face

- Lay him on his changing mat or next to you on the sofa
- Sit him up on your lap
- Hold him away from the warmth of your body while feeding
- Walk round the room with him while you are feeding.

For small and premature babies in particular, sucking is hard work and it is more difficult to keep them awake for feeds. Remember to try latex teats.

The secret life of a baby's wind

Locating your new baby's wind can be frustrating – for both you and him. You know there's a burp inside somewhere but it seems to be taking for ever to come out. In the meantime your baby is squirming in discomfort and is just as desperate to get that burp out. Newborn babies can take an age to wind so patience is required. Once a baby reaches about eight weeks burping becomes a more efficient operation.

Some people advise winding a baby halfway through a feed, but babies often object vociferously if milk is taken away before they have finished. Break a feed to wind only if your baby is clearly in discomfort – squirming, wriggling or crying.

If your baby doesn't produce a burp after a few minutes try laying him down. If he cries soon afterwards, the wind is probably working its way upwards; pick him up now and the wind may surface on its own. If, however hard you try, a burp just won't surface, don't panic; it will eventually work its way out at his other end.

(Premature and low-birthweight babies may take longer than a few minutes to wind, although in the first few weeks the contrary can also be true as they are sleepy and don't take in much air when feeding.)

During night feeding babies don't gulp as much wind because they are relaxed and sleepy. You may not need to wind at all.

If wind is a persistent problem, give your baby an ounce of cool boiled water half an hour before feeds. There are some over-the-counter remedies which can be used from newborn and can be very effective. They work by bringing together the small bubbles of air in a baby's tummy to make bigger bubbles that can be released more readily. For maximum effect it needs to be used before each feed and over several days.

At first you may find it hard to know whether a cry is caused by wind. Here's how to tell. The cry will be intermittent and screeching, followed by a high-pitched squeal and accompanied by squirming – and sometimes by a baby drawing his legs up to his tummy. His face may go red and he'll have a gurgling tummy.

(Colic usually starts in the first month and is distinctive because it will last for hours – see p. 197.)

Jo's tried-and-tested ways of burping a baby

The koala
Hold your baby over your shoulder, cradling his bottom with your hand. Pat his back gently.

The bottle
Lie your baby on your knees face up, feet towards you. Rub his tummy in a clockwise motion. (This follows the direction of the intestine and helps the trapped air come to the top.) Slowly bring him back up to the sitting position.

The handshake
Sit your baby on your lap at a right angle to you. Use one hand to support his chest and the other to pat his back

gently, starting at the bottom of the back and working your way up. Do this several times to work the air out.

The bear hug
Sit your baby on your lap but facing away from you. Put both your arms around his middle and gently rock from side to side.

The corkscrew
While your baby is sitting on your lap, either facing you or facing away from you, hold him around his middle with both hands and gently twist him from side to side.

When a burp seems well and truly stuck, a combination of some, or all, of these positions usually produces results. But exercise restraint or your baby may think he's on a funfair ride and start to feel sick. You will soon find out which one of these methods suits him best.

Sleep

Your baby's, that is . . .

Signs of tiredness

- Yawning
- Seeming to stare into the distance
- Rubbing the eyes (*for babies older than eight weeks*)
- Closing the eyes on and off
- Sucking the fingers or fist (this happens both when babies are tired and when they're hungry because they come to associate feeding with sleeping, so look for other signs of tiredness too)

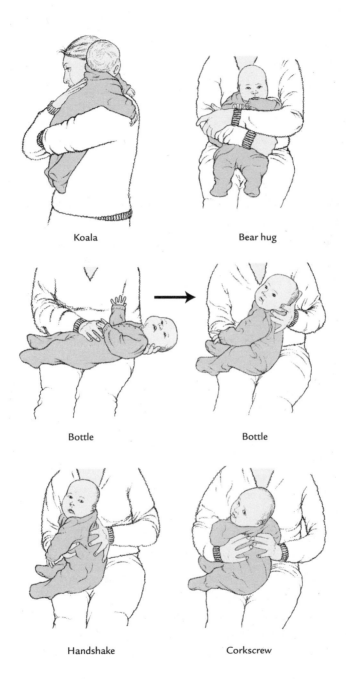

Koala

Bear hug

Bottle

Bottle

Handshake

Corkscrew

■ Crying – a cry of tiredness is a cry of frustration at the inability to fall asleep; it will start short and get louder and longer as a baby gets more tired.

Babies cannot stay awake for long periods or they get overtired and fractious. A newborn baby (up to six weeks old) cannot stay awake for longer than about one to one-and-a-half hours. From the age of six to ten weeks a baby can stay awake for about one and a half to two hours. Between ten weeks and four months this time becomes about two to three hours and between four and six months, three to four hours.

An overtired baby will find it hard to fall asleep; put your baby down for a nap before he gets overtired and he will sleep better.

Where is my baby going to sleep?

Your baby might love to sleep with you in your bed, and you might love the idea of having him there, but co-sleeping, as it is sometimes called, should really be avoided. It has been linked to cot death (also known as Sudden Infant Death Syndrome, SIDS), and it is strongly recommended that *a baby sleeps in his own cot.*

Both your baby and you benefit from his sleeping on his own. A baby who learns to sleep in his own bed will sleep better in the long run. (See chapter 7 on the importance of healthy sleep habits to your baby's development.) And there is no doubt that you will sleep better without close infant company and you need sleep too if you are to function at your best. According to Dr Richard Ferber, one of the leading experts on childhood sleep and author of *Solve Your Child's Sleep Problems*:

> We know for a fact that people sleep better alone in bed. Studies have shown that the movements and arousals of one person during the night stimulate others in the same bed to

have more frequent wakings and sleep-state changes, so they do not sleep as well.

And consider this: if you have decided to follow Jo's techniques because you want to get your baby to sleep through the night at an early age, *you will not manage it if your baby shares your bed.*

Your baby's cot should be made up in the 'feet to foot' position, with sheets and blankets halfway down the cot so your baby's feet lie towards the end board. This will make it hard for him to wriggle under the bedclothes.

Or you can use a sleeping bag once you stop swaddling your baby. Use a firm mattress and never use pillows or duvets for a baby under a year old.

The safest way for your baby to sleep is on his back. And you need to be sure that he does not overheat, which is very dangerous for a baby.

The ideal temperature for your baby's room is between 60° and 70°F: a thermostatically controlled heater may give you greater control over this than a central heating system. A good rule of thumb is that your baby should wear one more layer of clothes and bedclothes than you. A quilt is about the same as two blankets, so if you are wearing pyjamas under a quilt, he should have a vest, a sleepsuit, a sheet and a blanket.

If he is swaddled, this counts as a sheet.

If you are using a sleeping bag, follow the instructions as they have different 'tog' levels. To check whether your baby is too hot, feel his tummy and look for signs of sweating.

You can put a baby into a cot straight away but some parents like to use a moses basket for the first six weeks or so. If you opt to do this, prepare your baby for the move to his cot by putting him in it at some stage during the day as you potter round the room. He can get used to the new space while feeling secure in your presence. For a few days before the move, pop the moses basket inside the cot at night.

Daytime naps should take place either in a baby's rocker chair (tilted flat), his moses basket (but anywhere other than his bedroom, which is for night-time only), his pushchair if you want to get out of the house (see below), or his car seat in the car (but don't leave a baby under six months in a car seat for more than two hours at a time as it may be bad for his back). You don't need to put your baby in his cot for daytime naps until he has learned to sleep through the night or he may get confused about the difference between day and night.

If your baby is at home try to find a quiet room or a quiet corner for him to sleep, but don't worry about keeping background noise during naps too low or you'll soon find you have to tiptoe round him every time he snoozes. Try facing his rocker chair towards a wall to minimize distractions.

Swaddling your baby

'I swaddle all the babies I work with in the first six to eight weeks. I've noticed that it helps them to sleep better and when I come across babies who have had sleep problems at an early age it nearly always turns out that they weren't swaddled.

'I like to paint the following picture to explain to parents why their baby might need to be swaddled. Imagine he has spent nine months feeling secure in the womb where there are physical boundaries that he can feel all around him. Once he is born there are no "walls" around him and he feels as if he is standing on top of a cliff and about to fall at any moment. When you think about it like that you can see why it is so effective.

'I swaddle fully at night and half-swaddle – putting the sheet around a baby's shoulders loosely like a cocoon – during the day for naps.'
Jo

Babies are born with a number of reflexes: one is the 'startle reflex'. This happens when a baby is startled by a loud sound – it could even be his own cry – or by a sudden movement. He will extend his neck, throw out his arms and legs and then bring them back as if to cling on to something. This often happens as he is falling asleep and will wake him up with a jolt. Swaddling helps to counteract the reflex, thereby preventing it from waking up the baby. You don't have to swaddle, but recent research has backed up the view that it does help babies to sleep better.

You need a small lightweight cotton sheet for swaddling and should never use a blanket or anything thicker. A pram sheet is fine. You will be shown by your midwife how to swaddle your baby.

If at any time before six weeks you feel your baby is fighting his swaddling cloth, try to keep one of his arms out. Some babies seem to need to suck a fist or have a hand close to the face for comfort; this may be a throwback to their position in the womb. Observe your baby asleep to work out which fist he wants.

Once a baby reaches six to eight weeks he will start to stretch out and sleep in the 'starfish' position. This is the time to stop swaddling (and to take him out of a moses basket or his out-stretched arms will hit the sides and wake him).

At this stage you can half-swaddle him at night too, and

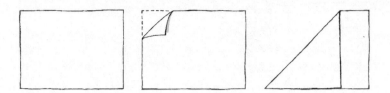

Take the shortest corner and fold over to the other side, so one side is thin and the other is wide

After folding sheet as shown...

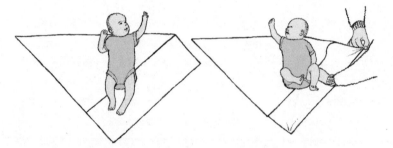

Put baby in centre of sheet

Take the widest piece, put baby's arm down by its side

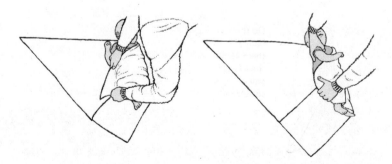

Fold over baby

Roll baby towards you and tuck the sheet under baby

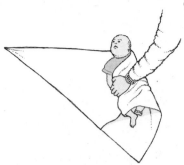

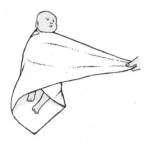

Take other side of sheet and put
baby's other arm by the side

Take sheet across baby

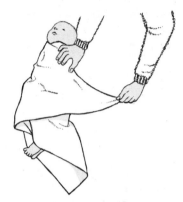

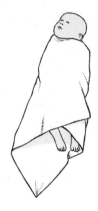

Roll over on to side and tuck sheet
under baby

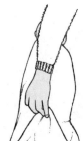

Half swaddle

Do the same but don't put
baby's arms by its side. Have
them up near face – bent at
the elbows – but with sheet
still cocooned around the
shoulders

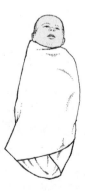

If there is enough sheet take the bottom
and tuck it in between the folds

Full swaddle

abandon swaddling altogether once he starts to try to wriggle free. Try replacing his swaddle with a sleeping bag. Sleeping bags avoid the problem of blankets falling off in the night – another cause of night waking.

How can I get my baby to sleep well?

In the first couple of weeks of a baby's life he is very sleepy – premature babies particularly so. This is helpful in that it gives mums a chance to recover from the birth, but it can also lull parents into thinking that they are either lucky to have a 'good' baby or that taking care of a newborn is not as difficult as it's cracked up to be. Babies must be woken for feeds during this period or they will not get enough milk and when they 'wake up' at two weeks they will be very hungry. But remember that a baby cannot stay awake for more than one to one and a half hours at this age (see p. 60).

The biggest impact you can have on your baby's long-term sleeping patterns can happen in the first two weeks, and following Jo's advice will make it easy for you to get your baby sleeping through the night by the time he is only a few weeks old. Chapters 7–10 will show you in detail how to achieve it, but you can lay the foundations now.

'I think babies are born with the ability to fall asleep on their own, but we parents and carers too often mess it up for them. We cuddle them in our arms as they fall asleep, let them doze on the breast, rock them to sleep when they are tired, or try to get them to sleep by pushing them in a buggy. But, although it is completely understandable, it doesn't help our babies.

'If your baby is going to learn to sleep well, you must

put him down awake, from the day he is born, so that he can do the falling asleep bit himself. Otherwise, he will not learn to fall asleep without being rocked, cuddled or given a breast.

'If you don't manage to do this in your baby's first weeks, don't panic. You can start at any stage – and of course you need to feel comfortable when you do – but as with so many things, the earlier you do it, the easier it will be for everyone.'

Jo

This is what you need to do:

1. Always lay your baby down for a sleep *awake*. If you see him falling asleep on the breast, nudge him awake gently and then lay him down awake. If you want to go out with him in the pushchair, wait – if you can – until he is asleep in the pushchair before leaving, so that he doesn't start to use motion as a way of helping him fall asleep. Try to do the same before car journeys.

   If your baby is so tired or fretful that he can't settle, rocking him in a pushchair indoors is a wonderful way to soothe him. Some babies find their pushchair the best place to nap. It is still possible to catch the moment he actually drifts off to sleep and stop rocking just before.

   The same applies to naps in his rocker chair. Rock it gently to settle an unsettled baby but stop before he falls asleep.

2. Start to differentiate between day and night for your baby as soon as you can. Please consult the advice in chapter 8 on bedtime rituals and night–day differentiation. Follow a bed-time ritual as soon as you feel comfortable and try to ensure

that your baby spends his night hours in a quiet darkened room. The advice in chapter 9 on stretching his night-time feeds can be started once a baby (healthy and born at term) reaches about two weeks.

3. Start a log of your baby's sleeping patterns through day and night as soon as you can. This will help you identify when he needs to sleep, particularly during the day, and will help you to put him down awake before he gets overtired. Babies who settle before they are overtired tend to sleep better; overtired babies find it hard to fall asleep. Your baby's sleep log will also help you when you put your baby in a routine, by showing you when he gets tired and needs to nap.

Coping with the onset of exhaustion

Yours, that is . . .

There comes a point soon after a baby arrives when piles of dirty washing, clothes to be ironed and layers of dust conspire to stress the calmest of new parents. You may know rationally that it doesn't matter if the house is messy, but emotionally you may find it hard to accept. Sometimes things can get on top of even the most organized new mum and, if you have no help to get you through, it can be tough (see chapter 13 on finding help).

Dads can ease the burden on their partners by doing a few things to lighten the load in addition (of course) to the shopping and cooking. Be encouraging to your partner even if you feel that it is you who really needs some praise. Don't underestimate the value of telling her she's doing brilliantly – whatever you think. (She might even return the compliment . . .)

Once you're back at work, phoning your partner regularly can help, as does telling her when you plan to be home – and sticking to it. Getting back in time for your baby's bath will be fun for you and a relief for mum. Whatever you do, don't say you need time to relax as soon as you walk through the front door; the days when you could do that are gone.

Sharing the night-time feeds is a help. You could do the late-night feed (using a bottle of formula or expressed milk) so your partner can rest before taking over in the middle of the night. You might also enjoy getting your baby up in the morning. This will allow your partner a little longer in bed and give you some time with your baby before you go to work.

Allocate an afternoon (or even just a couple of hours) every weekend for mum to be free to do her own thing and for you to be alone with your baby (without anyone looking over your shoulder).

Dads get exhausted too, though, and are not immune from the overwhelming emotions that come with having a new baby. They may also feel under intense pressure at work knowing that their partner is at home alone with a new baby. Colleagues may expect them to carry on as normal despite the fact that they are often tired. This is a time when both parents can feel stressed and need, somehow, to cut each other a little slack.

All of which is so much easier if you are both getting some sleep. And this need not be far away. One of the first steps towards achieving it is to put your baby into a feeding routine once he is between one and two weeks old.

3.

Why Routines are the Secret to Confident Parenting

'All new mums face a big decision some time soon after their baby is born: whether to put their baby on a routine or simply feed him on demand.

'I've looked after many babies over the years and I can categorically say that the best way to care for a new baby is to feed on a routine. I don't know a single baby who hasn't thrived, and I don't know a single mother who hasn't been won over too, once she has seen how easy a routine is to follow and how much her baby loves it. I've noticed time and again how mothers with babies on routines are always the most confident and the calmest mothers around.

'I am often called out to help mums who have spent several weeks feeding on demand and are finding it imposs-ible to cope with a grizzly, miserable baby who snacks all day and never sleeps for any length of time. These mums are at their wits' end and utterly exhausted. It usually takes only a few days before things change – for the better. The mums sometimes joke that I have exchanged their baby for a different one, the change is so drastic!

'But it comes as no surprise to me that a fretful and fussy baby can be transformed into a smiling contented one. As everything slots into place and he feels he can make sense of the world, it is as if the baby lets out a huge sigh of relief. Instead of snacking all day a routine-fed baby builds an appetite for regular "meals" and his tummy is full after eating and he feels satisfied. He begins to nap better during the day, sleep better at night and is less tired and cranky. And he feels secure and comforted by always knowing what is happening and when: babies crave certainty, including being sure when their next meal will turn up.

'The routine helps mums too. One mum told me she had shied away from the idea because she thought it meant being strict and disciplined – which she didn't think she could be. It took only twenty-four hours for her to confess, "I could not have been more wrong. The change it has made to my life is unbelievable. My baby and I are no longer in a mess." Her favourite phrase now is: "A routine is sanity."

'This chapter will tell you about the wonders of a routine for your baby (and for you . . .) and will give you some guidance on when and how you can start.'

Jo

'When my boys were four months someone told me, rather wistfully, that they seemed "like perfect babies". I had to smile because I knew they were really no different from any others. What they did have was a routine. And they loved it.

'They would nap happily at set times during the day and because they were always rested they were rarely grizzly. They slept through the night from three months and in the mornings would wake up cheerful. Regular feeds meant they ate well and heartily; routine feeding also meant I could pinpoint the reason for any crying: I knew when it was hunger and when it wasn't, so I could react quickly. As a first-time mum the confidence I gained from this was wonderful.

'There is no doubt in my mind that babies love routine. I saw it for myself. Now that my boys are toddlers they still love having predictability and structure in their lives and I am so glad I started early. The baby routines laid solid foundations for what came later.

'Nor is there any doubt in my mind that a routine makes life easier for parents. It did for me – and I don't think any mum should feel guilty about doing something for herself for once! After all, happy parents make good parents.'
Barbara

What is a routine?

A routine simply provides structure to your baby's day in a world where chaos could reign – if you let it. It sets out times for feeds, play time and naps (in that order) ensuring that a baby both drinks and sleeps enough during the day – after all, milk and sleep are the two most important things he needs. If the word routine conjures up images of a regimented approach to babycare, rest assured that nothing could be further from the truth.

The wonder of a routine is that it follows a baby's natural feeding and sleeping patterns, the patterns a baby might settle into spontaneously over time, but which he can achieve very quickly with a little help and guidance from you. Getting a routine started early in your baby's life simply speeds up the process.

Once a routine is established a baby will enjoy having regular meals and regular naps. He will feel secure and confident. Good sleeping patterns will soon follow and your baby will be better rested. Routine-fed babies really are happy babies.

Anyone can opt for a routine. Routines are easy to follow and are just as successful with breastfed as with bottle-fed babies. (Breastfeeding mums simply need to ensure that their milk supply is established and that their baby is latching on and drinking confidently before they begin.)

Perhaps most important of all, a routine is the surest way of achieving the Holy Grail of a baby's early months: SLEEPING THROUGH THE NIGHT. Having a baby on a routine means night-time sleep need not be a distant dream. It is a reality, achievable sooner than you had dared to hope.

If a baby sleeps, everyone benefits. Parents often comment how much happier their baby is once he starts to sleep through the night. Routines mean happy parents too: who could be happier than a parent who can also sleep through the night? And rested parents surely make better parents. Mothers (and fathers) find they enjoy working with a routine because it restores some order to their lives.

What is my alternative?

One way to demonstrate the wonders of routine is to consider its alternative, which is to feed a baby on demand. Mothers of new babies are usually advised by health professionals to demand-feed, and it does have the benefit of being straightforward and easy to understand. But if you think how you yourself might feel about it, you can just as easily understand why feeding your baby on a routine is so much more suitable.

Imagine your favourite snacks are chocolate and crisps, and you keep several bars and bags on the kitchen table. Whenever you feel peckish you help yourself – a little at a time, on and off, all day long. By the evening, all that nibbling means the last thing you fancy is a proper meal. Your appetite is wrecked, so you spend the evening nibbling yet more chocolate and crisps. By the time you go to bed you are probably still peckish, and if you aren't, you certainly will be in the middle of the night. Would you not, honestly, prefer to have had three good meals during the day, and to have built up a good appetite before enjoying them?

Your baby is no different. A baby who feeds on demand learns to snack and he will snack on and off on his favourite food all day long. Every time he is peckish he will ask to be fed. He will not be really hungry so he won't have a full feed and the little he takes won't last him long – so he will be peckish again quite soon after. He will never have the feeling of being truly ready for a proper meal, of having built up an appetite before it, and of having the satisfaction of a nice full tummy afterwards. Snacking becomes a habit. Snacking babies get exhausted. Overtired babies can find it hard to sleep. It is a horrible cycle.

It doesn't stop there. Snacking babies tend to drink more of the watery non-calorific foremilk from the breast, because they are never on the breast long enough to reach the more filling and nutritious hindmilk. This just adds to their cycle of feeling peckish, but never satisfied, all day long. (Frequent feeding can also exacerbate wind and may even increase the likelihood of colic.)

And babies who are fed on demand don't always demand. In the first few weeks of life babies are sleepy. They can sleep for long stretches without demanding to be fed, when what they need is a regular intake of milk. When they get past the sleepy stage, they can suddenly realize they are very hungry as they haven't been taking in enough milk.

And what about mum? Some mothers feed on demand as often as every hour; even, in extreme cases, every half an hour. After a few weeks of doing this round-the-clock any mother would be exhausted. Exhaustion and sleep deprivation are not to be taken lightly as they increase the chances of postnatal depression and put great pressure on relationships. Exhaustion is also the main reason mothers give up breastfeeding.

A pattern of feeding little and often can go on for months, and not just through the day. A baby will expect it to continue through the night too, both because he has become accustomed to it and because he is hungry from not having had enough milk during the day. *Frequent feeding makes it harder for a baby to sleep through the night.* This has been confirmed by research conducted by Dr Ian St James Roberts at the Thomas Coram Institute, part of the University of London's Institute of Child Education, published in January 2003. It showed that newborn babies who fed frequently were much more likely to have problems sleeping through the night by the age of twelve weeks than those who fed less frequently. It made no difference whether the babies were breast- or bottle-fed.

Routines really are the best option.

How routines give parents knowledge and understanding

> 'Having a routine was great for my baby, for me and for my husband. Before we started it my husband would come home and say, "What do we do with the baby now?" and I wouldn't know. Once we had a routine he knew what was happening and didn't have to ask all the time. He could take over the reins and look after his little girl all by himself, without me telling him what to do all the time. He was so much happier.'
> **Robin**

Your baby's routine is empowering because it gives you knowledge – and knowledge is a powerful tool. When your baby is on a routine you will always know when he is due to be fed, to sleep or to play. This will free you up to plan your days with some certainty that things will work out the way they were planned. It can feel very liberating.

For example, if you know that your baby always feeds at midday and then has a long nap, you can plan ahead to use that time to catch up on chores. If you want to get out of the house and take your baby with you, you can work out the best time to do so, after a feed maybe or during your baby's nap. You can even ask a friend, relative or babysitter to look after him, safe in the knowledge that you can tell them what needs doing and when; nothing need be left to chance. Other family members will also love knowing what is happening, particularly older children.

Here is a fictional but entirely realistic example of the way a routine is so helpful for parents, when compared with its alternative:

> wo mums with six-week-old babies arrange to meet for a coffee. Mum1 has her baby on a routine; Mum2 feeds on demand.
>
> Mum1 knows that her baby is due for a morning nap followed by a feed at 10.30 a.m. so she arranges to meet Mum2 at eleven, after her baby's feed. Mum2 is happy to meet at any time because she doesn't know when her baby will want to feed or sleep.
>
> Mum2's baby cries for a feed at 9.30. He isn't offered a morning nap afterwards because he doesn't seem tired. Mum2 and her baby leave the house at 10.45, but as they walk to the coffee shop the baby starts to cry for a feed again. As soon as they arrive Mum2 feeds him. He doesn't take much milk because he isn't very hungry, and he is now overtired because he hasn't slept all morning.
>
> Mum1 arrives at the coffee shop with a happy baby who has a full tummy after a satisfying feed and who has had a morning nap and is not overtired. At 11.30 she knows he is due for another nap, which he has in his pushchair. She lays the seat flat, turns the pushchair to the wall so her baby is not distracted,

rocks it a few times and her baby falls asleep five minutes later.

Mum2's baby's overtiredness means it takes her twenty minutes to rock him to sleep in his buggy. It is quite hard to talk to her friend . . . When he finally falls asleep, Mum2 is edgy because she doesn't know how long he will sleep. After all he didn't drink much before he slept so he may wake suddenly from hunger. So she orders a coffee quickly and leaves.

Mum1 orders a coffee and sits back to read the newspaper. She knows her baby isn't due for another feed until 2 p.m. and won't wake for another hour – so she can relax!

This is a real-life example:

'We did a trip to the office today, working around the routines so Mary was perfectly predictable and consequently utterly angelic. We planned it so we took her round the shops for a bit while she was having her pre-lunchtime snooze and then fed her in the café at 1 p.m. We then trotted off to the office. She was awake for a short while and then conked out until 4 p.m. so she could be handed around my colleagues while out cold and hugely admired. I felt your routine was such a blessing.'
Rebecca, mother of Mary, four weeks old

The final blessing is that the knowledge a routine brings you will help you to understand your baby better. What more can any new parent ask? Parents who demand-feed their babies tend to react to most of their babies' cries by feeding, while parents with routine-fed babies don't and therein lies the secret. A baby does not cry through hunger alone. There are many reasons he might cry (as you will see in chapter 5). Feeding him on a routine will help you to identify confidently which cries are from hunger and which are not. For a parent, that ability is invaluable.

*'Your routine gave me such peace of mind. My brain was so
scrambled in the early months, so it was great not to have to
go through a thousand questions of what might be up with
the baby every time he cried. It leaves room in your head to
enjoy the fun part. Angus fell into it much quicker than we
could have imagined. I think it was his natural pattern from
the beginning – we just didn't know about it.'*
Morag

Here in summary are the benefits of feeding on a routine.

	Routine-feeding	*Demand-feeding*
Baby's feeding	Regular meals ensure babies eat as much as they need and are satisfied after eating	Babies snack and are not satisfied. Newborns may sleep through mealtimes and not drink enough
Baby's well-being	Babies thrive on predictability and are calmer and less likely to have wind or colic	Potential for colic and/or fussiness
Sleep	Potential for good sleep patterns and sleeping through the night at an early age	Potential for unsettled sleep patterns
Breastfeeding	A mother who is not exhausted is likely to breastfeed longer	Can be exhausting for mums, which means they are more likely to give up breastfeeding

	Routine-feeding	*Demand-feeding*
Mum and dad	Parents know what is happening and when, so can plan around their routine	Parents may be inhibited by the unpredictability of a baby's feeding patterns
Leaving the baby with other people	If you leave your baby with someone else you can tell them what will happen and when so they will know what to do	You may find it hard to instruct carers because you can't tell them what will happen and when. They may not feel comfortable about this
Siblings	Mum can tell older siblings when they will get her time because she knows when her baby will feed and when he will sleep	Siblings may find it hard to accept that a baby gets attention from mum whenever he cries. Mum may be unable to tell them when she has time for them
Understanding your baby	Parents learn to work out why a baby is crying, and to react to those needs, so they gain greater confidence	Parents react to cries by feeding as they assume all cries are from hunger and so may fail to spot other problems

Now that you know this is the best way forward, it is time to show you how it's done.

When can we start a routine?

You can start a routine early – when your baby is between one and two weeks old, as long as he is over about 6lb in weight. This is the ideal time as babies who start at this age slip into a routine very easily. When they are this young they are still a little sleepy and will follow what you ask quite readily. At about two weeks you simply make small adjustments to your routine if you need to, to accommodate their new alertness.

If you start a routine at this stage and are breastfeeding you must be sure that your breastfeeding is established before you begin. Your baby should be latching on and taking a full feed every time he drinks, and not snacking on and off. A rough guide is that he needs to empty one full breast at every feed. You will get to know when your breast has been drained: it becomes soft to the touch. A one- to two-week-old breastfed baby should be taking enough milk to last him around two and a half to three hours.

All babies are different in how long they need to take a full feed: watch your baby and learn his individual pattern. (There are some guidelines on p. 86.) Whether they are bottle-fed or breastfed, until they are three or four weeks old all babies need a little extra encouragement to take a full feed.

If you are not ready to start a routine as early as the first couple of weeks, simply wait until you are. It is best to feel comfortable and confident when you begin. But try, if you can, to get going before your baby reaches six weeks. Any later and your baby will have got used to doing things in a certain way and it may take him a while to readjust. Don't be disheartened if you don't see immediate progress. Stick at it: consistency is the key. You may, of course, find that things fall into place more quickly than you dared hope . . .

> '*I put Joe on a routine when he was three months because I was exhausted from demand-feeding and from the broken nights. He never seemed to sleep in the day either and he would cry if he was put down for more than ten minutes.*
>
> '*The routine Jo showed me was miraculous. I knew when he would have his daytime naps and I developed the confidence to let him cry for a couple of minutes to help him settle himself. It only took a couple of days for things to fall into place.*
>
> '*I felt like a new woman and that I was back in control again. My husband is the biggest cynic around and was sceptical that it would work, but he was converted: he still can't believe it.*'
> **Julie**

Whenever you start, there is a routine to suit your baby: with seven to choose from you can't go wrong. You can follow the age/routine guidelines on p. 86 when making your choice, but better still, keep a log of your baby's feeding and sleeping patterns for between five and seven days beforehand and use it to help you match your baby's patterns with a routine.

Once you start the routines, stick closely to Jo's six secrets and you should find that everything else slots into place.

Jo's secrets to making a routine work

The first secret
is *always follow the order of events of the routines*: wake your baby, feed him, play with him, nap time. Don't worry if the exact timings don't go by the book, but do try to keep the sequence the same. Consistency is the key.

The second secret

is that *the first feed of the day should always be at the same time*, usually between 7 and 7.30.

The third secret

is that *bedtime, and the bedtime feed, should always be at the same time*, about twelve hours after your baby has woken up. If you are not convinced that it makes any difference when a baby goes to bed, think how debilitating jet lag can be. Chopping and changing your sleep times can be very wearing.

The fourth secret

is that *all the other timings are flexible* so you can relax about hitting them exactly. Any feed can take place up to fifteen minutes earlier or up to fifteen minutes later than the time it is due.

The fifth secret

is *always give yourself a minimum of seven days* before things slip into place. It may take less.

The sixth secret

is, if ever you find things slipping drastically and you feel your routine is falling apart, *don't give up*! Just start afresh the following morning.

Some tips before you start

- A newborn baby (up to six weeks old) cannot stay awake for longer than about one to one and a half hours without getting overtired and fractious. From the age of six to ten weeks a baby can stay awake for about one and a half to two hours. Between ten weeks and four months this time becomes about two to three hours and between four and six months, three to four hours. If your baby stays awake longer than these times, he will get overtired and find it hard to sleep. Make sure you put him down for a nap before he gets to that stage.

- Babies who are only a few weeks old may be reluctant to wake for feeds; this is normal. It is really important that you wake your baby for his feeds at the time he needs them and that he takes a full feed every time. Parents sometimes leave a baby to sleep for long stretches, which is what a newborn baby will often do. Unfortunately, this can begin a dangerous cycle where a baby sleeps so much during the day that he never drinks enough milk and ends up starving at night, when he will be wide awake with hunger. As babies get older they do start to wake more readily, but until that happens you will need to intervene. (There are ideas on how to do this on p. 51.)
- Changing nappies fifteen to twenty minutes before a feed helps to wake a baby up; it also means he is clean, dry and comfortable while having his meal.
- Keep a log of your baby's feed and especially his sleep patterns before you start the routine and continue to do so. Observing when your baby is sleepy will help you to settle him before he gets overtired and help him to nap better. The log will also help you to adapt the routines when and if you need to. For example, you might notice that your baby's morning nap gets shorter, which will probably be a sign that he is ready to do without it. A log will also enable you to monitor progress over time which can give you encouragement whenever you need it.

4.

The Daily Routines

'One of the key secrets to making a routine work is to make sure you, the parents, are comfortable – and confident – about following it.

'So I always stress to parents that:

- Your routine is not a dictator, but a guide
- Your routine is flexible and you can make adjustments if and when you need to. You can vary any of the times by fifteen minutes either way
- Your routine is chosen by you according to your baby's age and individual needs. All the routines are based on babies' natural feeding patterns at different stages of their early lives but as all babies are different, it will be up to you to decide exactly which routine suits your baby best.

'A routine should be one which makes everyone happy. This chapter will help you to choose your routine.'
Jo

There are seven routines to choose from, starting with Routine 1 – two-and-a-half-hourly feeds – up to Routine 7 where feeds are every four hours, but you will not necessarily work your way through all seven. These routines will serve you until your baby is around six months old, when he will be weaned on to solids.

Which routine do I choose?

'I usually put newborn babies on to a three-hourly routine (Routine 3) at around one to two weeks old. Sometimes mums prefer to feed a little more often, in which case they can start with Routine 1 or 2 (every two and a half or two and three-quarter hours) and move gradually to Routine 3. However, if a baby weighs less than 7 lb, I would always start with the two-and-a-half hourly routine, moving gradually to three-hourly feeding once the baby passes the 7 lb mark. The three-hourly routine is the most straightforward and seems to suit both babies and mums really well.

'When a bottle-fed baby gets to around eight weeks (sometimes a little earlier), I suggest stretching the feed by fifteen minutes, and then at three months I would stretch it further, until a four-hourly routine has been reached at about four to five months.

'I find that breastfed babies tend to stay on the three-hourly routine for longer and will usually not be ready to be stretched until around three months.

'Your goal is to be feeding four-hourly at around four to five months – but you don't *have* to reach that goal; be guided by what you think suits your baby best.'

Jo

Use the following tables to help you decide which routine you feel would be best for your baby. The tables include guidance on feeding quantities. Be guided too by the log of your baby's feeding and sleeping patterns. If you find after a week on one routine that it doesn't feel right, try another. Your aim is to have a baby who has an appetite and is ready for his feeds and able to take a full feed each time.

You will know when your baby is ready to be moved to another routine and have his feeds stretched: his age will guide you but so will his behaviour. You will notice that he is not as hungry at feeds and that is a sign that you can stretch them. Each time you do so you will be varying the feed times by only fifteen minutes and it should not take long for your baby to adapt.

To follow the routines you will also be helped by knowing approximately how much sleep your baby needs during a full day. Please remember though that because all babies are different the sleep table is only a guide. Your own observations of your baby's napping patterns will be just as helpful. It is really important to ensure that your baby does not sleep more than he needs during the day. Otherwise he will find it harder to sleep for a long stretch at night and be more likely to wake early in the morning. But don't assume that depriving him of daytime sleep will make him likely to sleep better. *Overtired babies find it hard to sleep.* That is why the sleep chart is so important.

All dates are for healthy babies born at term. If your baby was born prematurely please adjust for prematurity: be guided by your baby's weight.

Which routine? For breastfed babies

Babies below 7lb	*Routine 1:*	Amount:
	every 2½ hours	up to 20 minutes

Most small babies will be exhausted after sucking for 20 minutes on the breast; if yours is exhausted but still seems hungry, you might want to give him expressed milk from a bottle.

Many low-birthweight babies will have been in special care where they will have been fed every 3 hours. In this instance continue the 3-hourly routine but switch to a 2½-hourly routine if you feel your baby is finding it hard to last 3 hours between feeds. If your baby was sent home from the Special Care Baby Unit (SCBU) on a 4-hourly routine, you might be advised to revert to a 3-hourly routine or you may find you are feeding through the night for longer than you need.

2–4 weeks/7–9lb approx.	*Routine 1, 2 or 3:* every 2½–3 hours	Amount: 15–35 minutes

Most babies up to the age of four weeks will take only one breast. If your baby is still hungry after 25 minutes on the breast and you think he has emptied it, offer him the second for 10 minutes. This may happen around the three-week mark when babies have a growth spurt.

4–8 weeks/up to 11lb approx.	*Routine 3:* every 3–3¼ hours	Amount: 20–35 minutes

Your baby will still probably be getting his full feed from the first breast, but offer the second breast after 25 minutes if he is still hungry.

2–4 months/up to 14/15lb	*Routine 3, 4 or 5:* every 3–3½ hours	Amount: 20–30 minutes

By this stage your baby should be an expert breastfeeder so he will be feeding without getting too sleepy. He will also have a stronger suck so will be taking more milk in each feed, which is why the duration of feeding does not change noticeably from the early weeks. You will also find that your baby will want to move on to the second breast at most feeds. At first this will be for a short time, but will increase as he gets bigger.

4–6 months/15lb and up	*Routine 5, 6 or 7:* every 3½–4 hours	Amount: 15–25 minutes

Which routine? For formula-fed babies

Babies below 7lb	*Routine 3:* every 3 hours	Amount: approx. 2–3oz

Many low-birthweight babies will have been in special care where they will have been fed every 3 hours. In this instance continue the 3-hourly routine but switch to a 2½-hourly routine if you feel your baby is finding it hard to last 3 hours between feeds. If your baby was sent home from the Special Care Baby Unit (SCBU) on a 4-hourly routine, you might be advised to revert to a 3-hourly routine or you may find you are feeding through the night for longer than you need.

2–8 weeks/7 to 11lb	*Routine 3 or 4:* every 3–3¼ hours	Amount: 4–5oz
2–4 months/up to 14/15lb	*Routine 4, 5 or 6:* every 3¼–3¾ hours	Amount: 5–7oz
4–6 months/15lb and over	*Routine 6 or 7:* every 3¾–4 hours	Amount: 6–9oz

Do not give a baby 'hungry baby' formula unless he has taken 8oz at a feed and is still hungry.

How much sleep does my baby need?

Age	Daytime sleep	Number of naps	Night-time sleep	Total sleep
Low-birth-weight babies (under 7lb)	7–9 hours	6 – about 15 minutes after a feed has ended	10–12 hours Number of wakings: 2–3 (Up to 6½ lb your baby will need to be fed 3-hourly through the night)	19–21 hours
Newborn–4 weeks	5–7 hours	Around 4 or 5 – about 15 minutes after a feed has ended	10 hours Number of wakings: 2–3 (dream feed plus two others)	17–19 hours
4–12 weeks	4–6 hours	Around 3 or 4 Babies will stay awake longer after their feeds now	11–12 hours Number of wakings: 1–3 (dream feed plus one or two others)	16–18 hours
3–4 months	3–4 hours	3	12 hours Number of wakings: 0–1 (dream feed until dropped)	15–16 hours
4–6 months	2–4 hours	2	12 hours Number of wakings: 0	14–16 hours

What to do – a step-by-step guide

All seven routines are summarized later in this chapter, but to help you understand what happens at every stage, here is Routine 3 in detail. Simply transfer the information to the particular routine you choose.

07.00–07.15 Open the curtains and wake your baby (if he isn't already awake) with a cheery 'Good morning'. (Babies learn quickly to associate sounds with times of day; newborns' hearing is fully developed, unlike their eyesight.) Unswaddle him (if he's swaddled) and set the cot mobile going; the sound will become a familiar sign that the day has begun.

If he is still sleeping in a moses basket you could put him in his cot for a few minutes while you prepare for his nappy change, to help him get used to the bigger space.

This part of the day is one of the key pieces of the routine and should be stuck to as closely as possible. In order for your baby to have enough feeds during the day he needs to be awake for twelve hours before he goes to bed. If the time slips, your whole day will slide and bedtime will be delayed, making it harder for your baby to settle at night. You will reap the rewards of a regular start to the day very soon, even if you now feel that the last thing you want to do is to start getting up at seven every day if you're not used to it and are very tired.

If you need this time regularly to be later, make sure that all subsequent timings are moved by an equivalent amount.

Starting the day early means many dads can see their babies before they go to work, and can help mums with the feed.

Change your baby's nappy and take him out of the bedroom and/or downstairs.

07.15–07.30   Give your baby his first feed of the day.
Wind him.
Now it's play time.

08.00–09.00   Your baby will need a nap, starting some time between eight and nine o'clock. Don't worry how soon or how late it starts but be guided by the needs of babies of his age and by what you have observed of his sleep times; put him down before he is overtired.

09.30   Wake your baby (if he's not already awake), take him to his room to top 'n' tail him, change his nappy and dress him.

If you find it a struggle to wake your baby try:

- Tickling his chin
- Tickling a foot
- Blowing gently on his face
- Putting him down on his changing mat or another safe (but not overly-comfortable) surface.

10.00   Feed your baby. Remember that you don't have to stick to this time to the minute; you can bring it forward or delay it by up to fifteen minutes, if that suits you.

If you need to distract your baby while he is waiting for a feed, try walking round with him, showing him some toys or giving him a dummy.

When babies are still small (up to about four weeks) they often fall asleep during feeds. If this happens with your baby try:

- Tickling his chin
- Taking a foot out of his babygro and tickling it
- Using a baby wipe on his bare feet
- Blowing gently on his face
- Putting him down on the floor on his changing mat or on the sofa next to you
- Sitting your baby upright on your knee and at arm's length
- If you are bottle-feeding try walking round the room as you do so.

Wind your baby. (For the different techniques for winding a baby see p. 57.)
Play time again – see below.

11.00–12.00	Some time between eleven and twelve your baby will need to nap again, for about an hour.
12.30–12.45	Wake your baby (if he's not already awake) and change his nappy.
13.00	Feed and wind him. Play time as before.
14.30–15.30	He will need another nap around this time for about an hour.
15.30–15.45	Wake your baby (if he's not already awake) and change nappy.
16.00	Feed and wind him. Play time.

17.00–17.30   Your baby will probably need another short nap of fifteen to thirty minutes depending on his age, if he is to make it to bedtime without becoming overtired (which may prevent him from sleeping), but don't let him sleep past 17.30.

17.30   Wake your baby up.
Play time.

18.15   Once a baby reaches about four weeks you can introduce nappy-off time here. Nappy-off time is a godsend at a difficult time of day when babies are usually tired and grizzly.

Undress your baby's bottom half, take his nappy off and pop him on a changing mat on the floor. (You can use a disposable baby mat, washable blanket or towel.) Make sure the room is warm. Put an activity arch over him or some toys by his side.

Most babies love the liberating feeling of being out of a nappy and able to kick freely. It cheers them up and gives them some exercise. Getting air on a baby's bottom also helps keep nappy rash at bay.

Now it is time to start your baby's bedtime ritual, which is both the end of his day and an important part of helping him to wind down before the beginning of his night. (The bedtime ritual and its role in teaching a baby to settle and sleep through the night is explained in full in chapter 9.)

Bedtime ritual

18.30	Bath your baby. In the early weeks of his life you might prefer to top 'n' tail him (see p. 34). Dry him, put his nappy on and take him into the bedroom. Lay him on his changing mat and give him a massage. (Wait until your baby is at least four weeks old before doing this.) Use aqueous cream, baby massage oil or grapeseed oil.
19.00	Dress your baby in his night clothes, dim the lights and give him his feed. Try not to talk to him now or make eye contact. If he seems unsettled, calm him with a gentle sshhhhhh sound. This will help him to learn the cues for the approach of night-time. When he has finished feeding, wind him. You may have to spend about five minutes doing this as any wind left will make it hard for him to settle. Swaddle him (see p. 62) and lay him in his cot or moses basket, switch on his Slumber Bear or lullaby soother if you're using one and switch off the lights. Say goodnight and leave him in the darkened room. You may think it's daft to say goodnight to a tiny baby, but this will become part of his bedtime ritual and will be another cue for him that it is time to go to sleep. Your daily routine has ended. What you do now and for the rest of the night, until the day your baby settles and sleeps through, is explained in chapter 9.

What is play time?

You may, like many new parents, assume a baby is too young to 'play', but there are many things you can do to amuse and stimulate his developing brain. His focus at birth is only 8–12in (his eyesight will not reach maturity until about eight months) so he will love close eye-to-eye contact. His eyes will also be picking out high-contrast colours.

You could place your baby on a mat next to some black, white and red toys or books, put him in a baby carrier as you wander round the house, or pop him in his rocker chair with a brightly coloured activity arch over the top. Some mums put the chair in front of the washing machine or in front of a window for amusement.

Hearing music will interest him. In summer your baby could sit outside and listen to the sounds around him.

Don't forget that babies get bored after a while.

If you have older children who need to prepare for nursery or school, let your baby sit in the room with all of you and watch and listen.

It is very important that there is a break between your baby's feed and his nap because if he falls asleep too soon after his feed he will learn to associate feeding with sleeping and not learn to settle himself to sleep without it. Hence the importance of play time. It needs to be at least fifteen minutes long.

Where do naps take place?

Naps are best not taken in the cot until a baby is sleeping through the night. Taking daytime naps in the cot may confuse him and hinder your efforts at teaching him the difference between night and day. So put him in his rocker chair, tilt it so it is flat, cover him in a sheet or loosely swaddle him with his arms out if he is still under about six weeks. Put the chair in a quiet corner or in a quiet room, facing away from activity or facing a wall. If your baby struggles to nod off rock the chair a little to help him. If your baby is overtired and really struggling, give him a dummy but always use this as a last, rather than a first, resort. Don't rock him to sleep or he will want to be rocked every time.

Although it is good to find somewhere quiet for him, don't start tiptoeing around or whispering or he will never learn to nap through the inevitable hubbub of daytime. You could, if you want, play some soothing music in the background. If you have the television on, that's fine, but keep the sound low.

If you have other children or toddlers, you may want to put your baby in the nursery or another room, away from 'helpful' siblings.

When your baby's sleep patterns are well established and he's sleeping at night – at around three to four months, introduce the cot for daytime naps (see p. 134).

If you have a school or nursery run to do between eight and nine, or need to get out of the house during any of your baby's nap times during the day, take him and let him have his morning sleep in the buggy or the car. But a word of caution: babies who fall asleep regularly to motion find it harder to settle to sleep at night when the motion is not there. Try to settle your baby to sleep in his pushchair or car seat before you leave. If he needs help, rock the buggy gently or wheel it a few paces back and forth, but always stop before he falls asleep so that he falls asleep on his own and without the motion to help him.

Here now are the routines. Use the 'detailed routine' to fill in any information you need.

Please remember that the timings of feeds are guidelines: they are flexible and you can feed your baby fifteen minutes before or after any of the suggested times. The timings of naps are also guidelines. The exact amount your baby will sleep – and when – will depend on your baby's age and his own particular needs. Be guided by the sleep chart on p. 89 and keep a log of your baby's sleep patterns to help you find your baby's optimum nap times.

Remember to stick to the order:

- Wake
- Change nappy
- Feed
- Play
- Sleep.

'Please take it from me – these routines are easy to follow and really flexible. They aren't the Ten Commandments so you needn't feel that if you don't follow everything to the letter they won't work.

'Nor do you need to sit at home watching the clock. Quite the opposite. Once my boys were on a routine I was able to get out of the house more because I knew what they (and I) were doing and when.'
Barbara

The Routines

Routine 1

The two-and-a-half-hourly routine is designed for small babies who are underweight, and can be used until they reach 7lb. Once they reach that weight they can move towards a three-hourly routine.

Even if your baby is a healthy weight at birth you may want to start with this routine if you and your baby find it more comfortable. Then move towards the three-hourly routine as soon as you and your baby are ready – usually by about two to three weeks.

Tiny babies will be very sleepy through the day and you may struggle to make your baby take his feeds. You must persist as he needs his daily intake of milk.

Try to make sure that play time is always fifteen minutes. This can be hard when babies are tiny, but persevere.

The last two feeds of the day have only a two-hour gap between them. This helps to ensure that a baby is well fed before going to bed, when he may be so tired at this young age that he can't take a full feed.

Please note that the times and durations of your baby's naps will vary from baby to baby and depend on his age and how quickly he feeds.

Routine 1

2½ hourly	Daytime feeds: 6	Naps: 5
07.00	'Good morning!' Wake baby (if not awake) and change nappy, bring him downstairs	
07.00–07.15	Feed Play time Nap (starting *around* 08.00)	
09.15	Wake baby (if not awake) and change nappy Top 'n' tail him and dress	
09.30	Feed Play time Nap (starting *around* 10.00–10.15)	
11.45	Wake baby (if not awake) and change nappy	

Routine 1 *contd.*

2½ hourly	Daytime feeds: 6	Naps: 5
12.00	Feed Play time Nap (starting *around* 12.45–13.00)	
14.15	Wake baby (if not awake) and change nappy	
14.30	Feed Play time Nap (starting *around* 15.15–15.30)	
16.45	Wake baby (if not awake) but you don't need to change his nappy as it's close to bedtime	
17.00	Feed and put down for a nap straight away; no need for play time as baby will be very sleepy	
17.30	Short nap but don't let your baby sleep past 18.00	
18.00	Wake baby (if not awake) Play time	
18.15	Bath or top 'n' tail Massage in baby's room Dress in night clothes	
19.00–19.15	Feed Lights low, no talking 'Night night!' Switch off the light.	

Routine 2

The two-and-three-quarter-hourly routine will be used for small babies or newborns who started on Routine 1 but are now ready to have their feeds stretched. You will probably not stay on this routine for more than a week or two as your goal is to get to the three-hourly routine.

Because a twelve-hour day doesn't divide neatly into two-and-three-quarter-hour segments there is a reduced feed late in the afternoon to bridge the gap that inevitably arises. Although this is not two and three-quarter hours after the previous feed, it helps to ensure that a baby is well fed before going to bed, when he may be so tired at this young age that he can't take a full feed.

Please note that the times and durations of your baby's naps will vary from baby to baby and depend on his age and how quickly he feeds.

Routine 2

2¾ hourly	Daytime feeds: 5 + 1 reduced feed Naps: 5
07.00	'Good morning!' Wake baby (if not awake) and change nappy, bring him downstairs
07.00–07.15	Feed Play time Nap (starting *around* 08.00)
09.30	Wake baby (if not awake) and change nappy Top 'n' tail him and dress

Routine 2 *contd.*

2¾ hourly	Daytime feeds: 5 + 1 reduced feed	Naps: 5
09.45	Feed Play time Nap (starting *around* 10.45)	
12.15	Wake baby (if not awake) and change nappy	
12.30	Feed Play time Nap (starting *around* 13.30)	
15.00	Wake baby (if not awake) and change nappy	
15.15	Feed Play time Nap (starting *around* 16.15)	
17.15	Wake baby (if not awake), but you don't need to change his nappy as it's close to bedtime	
17.30	Reduced feed (to get baby through to bedtime feed – half the amount you would usually give) and put down for a nap straight away. Play time not needed	
17.45	Short nap if he needs it, but don't let him sleep past 18.00	
18.00	Wake baby (if not awake) Play time	

Routine 2 *contd.*

2¾ hourly	Daytime feeds: 5 + 1 reduced feed	Naps: 5
18.15	Bath or top 'n' tail Massage in baby's room Dress in night clothes	
19.00–19.15	Feed Lights low, no talking 'Night night!' Switch off the light.	

Routine 3

This routine is the most straightforward and the one that most babies will start on. Babies born at a healthy birthweight will usually adjust to it very easily, whether breast- or bottle-fed. Mums find it convenient too.

Breastfed babies will probably stay on this routine until they are about three months old.

Bottle-fed babies will probably be ready to move on from this routine to the next when they are about two months old.

Please note that the times and durations of your baby's naps will vary from baby to baby and depend on his age and how quickly he feeds.

Routine 3

3 hourly	Day time feeds: 5	Naps: 4
07.00	'Good morning!' Wake baby (if not awake) and change nappy, bring him downstairs	

Routine 3 *contd.*

3 hourly	Day time feeds: 5	Naps: 4
07.00–07.15	Feed Play time Nap (starting *around* 08.30)	
09.45	Wake baby (if not awake) and change nappy Top 'n' tail him and dress	
10.00	Feed Play time Nap (starting *around* 11.00)	
12.45	Wake baby (if not awake) and change nappy	
13.00	Feed Play time Nap (starting *around* 14.00)	
15.45	Wake baby (if not awake) and change nappy	
16.00	Feed Play time	
17.00	Short nap	
17.30	Wake baby (if not awake) Play time	
18.15	Nappy-off time (after four weeks) Bath Massage in baby's room Dress in night clothes	

Routine 3 *contd.*

3 hourly	Day time feeds: 5	Naps: 4
19.00–19.15	Feed Lights low, no talking 'Night night!' Switch off the light.	

Routine 4

Once you feel your baby is ready to move on from Routine 3 you can try this routine.

Because a twelve-hour day doesn't divide neatly into three-and-a-quarter-hour segments there is a reduced feed late in the afternoon to bridge the gap that inevitably arises.

Please note that the times and durations of your baby's naps will vary from baby to baby and depend on his age and how quickly he feeds.

Routine 4

3¼ hourly	Daytime feeds: 5	Naps: 4
07.00	'Good morning!' Wake baby (if not awake) and change nappy, bring him downstairs	
07.00–07.15	Feed Play time Nap (starting *around* 09.15)	
10.00	Wake baby (if not awake) and change nappy Top 'n' tail him and dress	

Routine 4 *contd.*

3¼ hourly	Daytime feeds: 5	Naps: 4
10.15	Feed Play time Nap (starting *around* 11.30)	
13.15	Wake baby (if not awake) and change nappy	
13.30	Feed Play time Nap (starting *around* 1500)	
16.00	Wake baby (if not awake) and change nappy	
16.45	Reduced feed (about three-quarters of a normal feed) Play time	
17.00	Short nap	
17.30	Wake baby (if not awake) Play time	
18.15	Nappy-off time Bath Massage in baby's room Dress in night clothes	
19.00–19.15	Feed Lights low, no talking 'Night night!' Switch off the light.	

Routine 5

Once you feel your baby is ready to move on from Routine 4 you can try this routine.

Because a twelve-hour day doesn't divide neatly into three-and-a-half-hour segments there is a reduced feed late in the afternoon to bridge the gap that inevitably arises.

Please note that the times and durations of your baby's naps will vary from baby to baby and depend on his age and how quickly he feeds.

Routine 5

3½ hourly	Daytime feeds: 4 + 1 reduced feed Naps: 3
07.00	'Good morning!' Wake baby (if not awake) and change nappy, bring him downstairs
07.00–7.15	Feed Play time Nap (starting *around* 09.15)
10.15	Wake baby (if not awake) and change nappy Top 'n' tail him and dress
10.30	Feed Play time Nap (starting *around* 12.00)
13.30	Wake baby (if not awake) and change nappy
14.00	Feed Play time Nap (starting *around* 15.30)

Routine 5 *contd.*

3½ hourly	Daytime feeds: 4 + 1 reduced feed Naps: 3
16.00	Wake baby (if not awake) and change nappy Play time
17.30	Reduced feed (half normal amount) Play time
17.45	Short nap for younger babies if needed
18.15	Nappy-off time Bath Massage in baby's room Dress in night clothes
19.00–19.15	Feed Lights low, no talking 'Night night!' Switch off the light.

Routine 6

This routine will help you to work towards feeding four-hourly. As you are now so close to feeding four-hourly – which is an easy routine to follow – you may not want to stay on this routine for long.

Because a twelve-hour day doesn't divide neatly into three-and-three-quarter-hour segments there is a reduced feed late in the afternoon to bridge the gap that inevitably arises.

Please note that the times and durations of your baby's naps will vary from baby to baby and depend on his age and how quickly he feeds.

Routine 6

3¾ hourly	Daytime feeds: 4 + 1 reduced feed Naps: 3
07.00	'Good morning!' Wake baby (if not awake) and change nappy, bring him downstairs
07.15	Feed Play time Nap (starting *around* 09.30)
10.30	Wake baby (if not awake) and change nappy Top 'n' tail him and dress
10.45	Feed Play time Nap (starting *around* 12.15)
14.15	Wake baby (if not awake) and change nappy
14.30	Feed Play time Nap (starting *around* 16.00)
16.30	Wake baby (if not awake) and change nappy
17.30	Reduced feed (half the usual amount)
17.45	Short nap for younger babies if needed Play time
18.15	Nappy-off time Bath Massage in baby's room Dress in night clothes

Routine 6 contd.

3¾ hourly	Daytime feeds: 4 + 1 reduced feed	Naps: 3

19.00–19.15	Feed
	Lights low, no talking
	'Night night!' Switch off the light.

Routine 7

This routine usually suits babies between four and six months old. It is a very easy routine to follow.

Please note that the times and durations of your baby's naps will vary from baby to baby and depend on his age and how quickly he feeds.

Routine 7

4 hourly	Daytime feeds: 4	Naps: 2

07.00	'Good morning!'
	Wake baby (if not awake) and change nappy, bring him downstairs

07.15	Feed
	Play time
	Nap (starting *around* 09.45)

10.45	Wake baby (if not awake) and change nappy
	Top 'n' tail him and dress (you can of course do this earlier in the day now that your baby's morning nap is later)

Routine 7 contd.

4 hourly	Daytime feeds: 4	Naps: 2
11.00	Feed Play time Nap (starting *around* 12.30)	
14.45	Wake baby (if not awake) and change nappy	
15.00	Feed Play time If your baby still seems tired he could have a short nap *around* 16.00 but he should soon be ready to drop this nap	
18.15	Nappy-off time Bath Massage in baby's room Dress in night clothes	
19.00–19.15	Feed Lights low, no talking 'Night night!' Switch off the light.	

If you come across problems in implementing the routines chapter 6 will help you get round them.

5.

The Secret to Knowing Why Your Baby is Crying

'There is nothing more baffling, perplexing and alarming than your own baby's cry – especially if you don't know the cause. Nature must have designed baby cries to bring maximum stress and worry to parents.

'When a baby cries, people expect mothers to know the reason, assuming maternal instinct can tell you. But it isn't that straightforward . . . Many of us need time to get to know and understand our babies before we learn to pinpoint quickly what is troubling them.

'In the first few weeks after my boys were born I was clueless (and stressed) when they cried – and they did their fair share. Jo told me that (other than illness) there were six key reasons why a baby cries and that we could quickly work through the list. Most people assume that a baby cries from hunger, but not every cry is a hunger cry. And if your baby is on a feeding routine you can very quickly identify or eliminate hunger as a reason.

'Understanding this transformed my understanding of my babies.

'The checklist that follows doesn't mean you should ever ignore your instincts, but when your baby cries it really will help to remove some of the mystery and get you closer, faster to working out what to do.

'I gave it to a friend. She got her husband to use it so he didn't have to ring her every five minutes whenever she left him with the baby . . .'
Barbara

Why is my baby crying?

1

Is it close to his feed time?
Does he show signs of hunger (rooting, head-butting your shoulder, sucking eagerly on your finger or clothing, pushing his fingers into his mouth, restlessness, grunting, opening his mouth wide and crying; are his cries short and sharp or does he shake his head in frustration if you give him a dummy)?

YES

He's hungry.
Distract him for a bit or feed him if it is time for a feed.

NO?

2

When did he sleep last?
Has he been awake for:

■ *Longer than one to one and a half hours if he is under six weeks?*
■ *Longer than one and a half to two hours if he is six to ten weeks?*

- *Longer than two to three hours if he is between ten weeks and four months?*
- *Longer than three to four hours if he is between four and six months?*

YES

He's tired — put him down for a nap.

NO?

3

Is he kicking his legs?

YES

He may have wind.

EITHER

- *Is he also writhing?*
- *Is there silence followed by a high scream?*
- *Is it late in the afternoon or early evening?*

YES

He may have colic.

OR

Is he also making straining noises?

YES

He may have constipation.

NO?

4

Is his nappy very wet or dirty?
Have a peek or a sniff.

YES

Change his nappy.

NO?

5

Has he been left alone or had the same toys to play
with for more than fifteen to thirty minutes?

YES

He's bored! Try a change of scenery or play with him.

NO?

6

When you feel his tummy is it . . .
Hot?

YES

Check his temperature. If he is over-heating, remove
a layer of clothing. If the temperature doesn't come
down, investigate further.

OR
Cold?

YES

Put on another layer of clothing.

If you cannot identify the reason for your baby's crying or if it is persistent, you should always seek medical advice.

6.

Problem-solving During the Day

'I want my routines to make parents feel comfortable not just when things are going well, but also when things don't go according to plan – and sometimes they don't. You and your baby will have ups and downs, and days when things are easier than others; it is quite normal if you, your baby and his routine take a knock at times. Every baby I have worked with has gone through phases when things have been easy and phases when things have been difficult.

'I have never expected miracles of anyone, or of any baby. So this chapter covers (I hope) most of the problems you're likely to face, and it comes with a promise that simple solutions are at hand.'

Jo

'When my boys were three months old I took them to a friend's birthday party and over the course of the afternoon several people commented on how calm and happy they seemed to be. One mum even asked jokingly whether they ever cried. I told her they usually grumbled for a few minutes before their feeds, which they promptly went on to do; they settled happily afterwards. I could hardly believe it, but despite having two small babies to look after, I had a stress-free and enjoyable party.

'I got such peace of mind from having a routine. One of the best things was the knowledge that when there were hitches or problems it didn't automatically mean I was doing anything wrong. I realized it was part and parcel of having a baby and what I had to do was look for solutions.

'There is an answer to most things and anyone following a routine with their baby will find the following guide a precious resource – and a comfort at times of stress.'
Barbara

The first six weeks . . .

What if . . .

My baby was born prematurely at thirty-five weeks and was in special care for two weeks. She is now at home weighing just 6lb. I find that breastfeeding takes an hour and a half as she feeds so slowly. Then we sleep for an hour before starting all over again.

A small baby like yours will be exhausted from sucking on the breast after only thirty minutes. If she is on the breast for an hour and a half she will be too tired to suck more than on and off and may not get all the milk she needs. She may even start to lose weight, which will be very worrying.

Until she is stronger (once she reaches about 7lb) you might limit her breastfeeds to thirty minutes and then 'top her up' with expressed milk from a bottle (use a latex teat which is easier for small babies to suck on). As long as your breastfeeding is established (which it clearly is) you shouldn't worry about nipple/teat confusion (see p. 52). Take the extra precaution at the beginning of a bottle-feed of rubbing the teat along your baby's lips until she opens her mouth rather than pushing the teat into her mouth without her having to work for it. This will stop her from getting lazy and encourage her to open her mouth for milk, which is what she needs to do when she feeds from the breast.

You could also change her nappy in the middle of a feed to keep her alert and more able to concentrate on feeding.

I have been observing the way my ten-day-old baby feeds and sleeps but I can see no pattern emerging whatsoever. I've heard that babies do slip into their own pattern so should I wait until he does so, before starting a routine?

With most babies, a sleeping pattern usually emerges in a few weeks but this happens less frequently with feeding. Some babies will feed erratically at first, and continue to do so for many weeks if not months. That's why they need to be guided into a routine. If there's no pattern to your baby's feeding, try putting him on Routine 3, the three-hourly routine, and see how he takes to it. If the gaps between feeds seem too long and he seems very hungry, try Routine 1 for a few days, before working gradually towards Routine 3.

My one-week-old baby falls asleep in mid-feed.

Newborn babies are very sleepy in the first two or three weeks. It is really important that they take their feeds or they may not get their full nutritional requirements during the day. That can mean a hard night when they wake frequently to make up for it. It's also a good idea for them to start to realize that the 'snack-bar' is not going to be open for them twenty-four hours a day or they may turn into persistent snackers, which is no fun for anyone.

Remember to change your baby's nappy before a feed to help him wake up. After that you could stroke his chin, blow gently on his face or undo the bottom of his babygro, take his foot out and tickle it. Sitting a baby upright on your knee is very effective. You could also play some music while you're feeding. If none of this works, put your baby on his changing mat, or lay him (safely) on the sofa. If you are bottle-feeding, try holding your baby in front of you but at a slight distance from your body. Babies can be lulled into sleepiness when held so this should wake him up. Walking around while feeding is surprisingly effective at getting a baby to pay attention to his feed.

If your baby hasn't taken his full feed an hour after you started it's time to stop. (If he protests, try giving him a dummy.) Your baby will be exhausted from sucking for such a long time, and at the next feed will be hungry and take more. This pattern will eventually improve and he'll take a full feed every time.

Some babies are very sleepy in the morning for two or three weeks after the birth. If you find this is making things difficult, you could express your milk and give this feed by bottle.

Feeding will get easier as the weeks go by.

My ten-day-old baby is crying even though he had a feed half an hour ago.
In the first two or three weeks of life babies can stay awake only for about an hour at a time. Your baby is probably tired and wants to sleep. Put him down for a nap.

My two-week-old baby is breastfeeding for one to one and a half hours at a time and it's exhausting me, but when I take him off the breast he screams.
Newborn babies usually get enough milk for a full feed in around twenty to thirty minutes (see chart on p. 87), but some babies take longer and some are quicker. Some suck consistently while others suck on and off; this determines how long a baby takes to feed. (As they get older, babies drain the breast more quickly. A baby of three months, for example, will usually get his feed in about twenty minutes.)

Once your baby has taken his full feed he is probably sucking for comfort, which can be exhausting for you and may give you sore nipples. He cannot be drinking consistently for an hour and a half or he would burst. You need to work out when the feeding finishes and the comfort sucking begins, and give him a dummy to satisfy his desire to keep sucking.

Try to limit feeds to forty-five minutes, and never go on for more than an hour; any more than that and your baby will be exhausted. You could offer thirty minutes on one breast and then ten to fifteen minutes on the other. Babies under about four weeks will be really tired after just thirty minutes of sucking. If you think your baby is too tired to finish his feed, you could give him an ounce or two of expressed milk from a bottle. (Sucking from a bottle is less tiring.) Reduce the amount you give by bottle gradually as your baby's sucking gets stronger.

Your baby may be screaming because he hasn't had a full feed as he has been sucking only intermittently. This can be a vicious circle. Drinking a little at a time means your baby never drains the breast and the breast never gets the chance to fill up. Your baby then never has the chance to have a full feed so is frequently hungry and sucks again, only to find there's not enough to satisfy him. If you are feeding frequently, you need to lengthen the gaps between feeds so he does get hungry and will start to take a full feed. Your aim is to get him on track for a routine that suits him. It may take a couple of days to adjust but it will happen.

If your baby is latched on properly, has drained the breast and isn't helped by a dummy it could be that he is overtired. Look at his sleep patterns and see if he is getting enough sleep. Babies who are very tired sometimes want the comfort of the breast to help them fall asleep, but this is not a good habit to get into as they may start to associate feeding with sleeping and think they cannot fall asleep without the breast to help them.

My two-week-old baby screams when I change his nappy.
Some babies love having their nappies changed and others hate
it; they feel uncomfortable having their skin exposed. If your
baby hates it, try putting cartoon stickers or black and white
photos on the wall next to the changing mat, or a mobile above
it. (You can cut photos out of magazines or draw some bold
black shapes on paper.)

Reassure your baby by playing the same music every time you
change his nappy – this could come from his mobile or a toy.

Babies usually learn to love nappy changes because of the
concentrated attention and eye-to-eye contact they get from mum
or dad, and they give parents some of their most rewarding smiles
at this time. You may even begin to use the changing mat as a
place to put your baby to cheer him up when he's cranky.

*My two-week-old baby sleeps happily for four to five hours during
the day. I don't understand why I should wake her to feed.*
Many parents are tempted to let a newborn baby sleep for long
stretches during the day. It does, after all, give them a chance to
catch up with chores or to rest, and they may have been told by
well-meaning friends or relatives to 'never wake a sleeping baby'.
But babies need to drink milk during the day and the only way
they can do this is if they are awake, so you must try to wake
your baby when her feeds are due. Otherwise you will follow the
path that well-meaning friends or relatives might not have told
you about, and find that your baby is awake all night through
hunger.

You may also find that your breasts have not been stimulated
sufficiently in the first few weeks because your baby has been
sleepy.

*My three-week-old baby hates nappy-off time and hates her
massage. Do I have to do them as part of the routine?*
Of course you don't. You and your baby should feel comfortable
with what you do and if there are things that don't work for you,
then give them a miss. Nappy-off time is best started once a baby
reaches four weeks so your baby may still not be ready. She may
also be a little young to enjoy a massage; try again in a couple of
weeks and see if she responds then. It's worth persisting because
babies usually love nappy-off time, and massages can be one of
the most fun parts of the day.

*My three-week-old baby won't stay awake for long after his feeds
and so we don't get much play time.*
Once your baby is about six weeks old he will become much
more alert during the day and you won't find it as hard to keep
him awake. So don't worry too much. Your goal at this stage is
to have your baby awake for around fifteen minutes before each
feed and fifteen minutes after (play time), so he has a spell of at
least an hour of being alert and awake, every three hours or so. If
you find this a struggle at first, wake your baby a little earlier and
reduce his play time. Remember that it's important not to let
him fall asleep immediately after a feed or he may start to associate
feeding with sleeping and come to depend on a feed to help him
fall asleep.

*My three-week-old baby suddenly seems to be extra hungry. Is this
normal?*
It is normal for babies to get very hungry when they're going
through growth spurts. Babies have growth spurts around day
six, day twelve, three weeks and six weeks, and it sounds as if that
is what is happening with your baby. (The growth spurts will
continue every few weeks after that.) You may need to offer him
the second breast at each feed, or an ounce of extra milk (formula

or expressed milk). Or you could try using an earlier routine (reducing the gaps between feeds by fifteen minutes) for two days and your milk supply will increase – then revert to the routine you were on.

I can't wake my three-week-old baby in order to feed him when you say I should.

That's why it can be a good idea to change your baby's nappy about fifteen minutes before a feed as this will help to wake him up and ensure that he's fully alert for his feed. Talk to your baby while you're doing it to help rouse him. You could also try tickling him under the chin, blowing gently on his face, undoing the bottom of his sleepsuit and pulling a foot out to tickle. Sitting your baby upright on your knee is also effective.

In the first couple of weeks of life babies are very sleepy and it may feel strange to be waking a baby, but at around four weeks of age, babies fed on a routine often start to wake automatically before their feeds as they get to know what's happening and when.

My baby is four weeks old and I am breastfeeding but I have no idea whether my baby is taking a full feed as he cries again an hour later.

Are you sure your baby is latching on properly? You may feel a tingling sensation which is the let-down reflex and that means your milk has started to flow. Look at your baby's throat and you should be able to see his swallows if he is drinking consistently. Your breast will feel softer when it is emptied.

If you think he is taking a full feed, look for other reasons he might be crying. He may not be hungry, but tired and crying for the breast to help him sleep. Try putting him down for a sleep, and give him a dummy if he has problems settling.

My four-week-old baby doesn't want his full feed.

In the first few weeks babies are sleepy, which can make them fussy about feeding. This will go in time. You can't force your baby to drink his milk, but at the same time you don't want him to get hungry again thirty minutes after the feed has finished.

If your baby is bottle-fed try to 'wiggle' the bottle in his mouth and pull the teat as if you are taking it away. Babies sometimes drink better if you stand up and walk around with them while feeding; it may sound strange but this does work.

A breastfed baby may need to be removed from the warmth and comfort of being snuggled against you, which can make him sleepy. Pop him on his changing mat or change his nappy to wake him up.

Once your baby is over six weeks old you can start to think about moving his feed on by fifteen minutes (moving to the next routine) and it's possible that he's already showing you he is ready for this. Try it for a couple of days and see if it makes him keener on his milk.

I'm worried that I'm not supplying enough breastmilk for my baby who is six weeks old.

Lots of mothers worry about this however old their baby is. If you need to put your mind at rest, express from both breasts half an hour before a feed and see how much you're producing. Remember that a breast pump isn't as efficient as your baby at draining the breast, so your baby will be getting slightly more.

A quick and simple rule of thumb is that if your baby is producing about six wet nappies a day and one dirty one and is putting on weight – 6–8 oz a week – then you're doing a great job.

If you feel you need to build up your milk supply you could use the following plan as a guide to help you. Eating well and getting as much rest as you can are essential. You should also aim to drink about 4 pints of water a day.

Building up your milk supply

Days 1–3

---

7 a.m.   Breastfeed, express from both breasts.

10 a.m.   Breastfeed, express from both breasts.

4 p.m.   Breastfeed, express from both breasts.

10 p.m.   Express from both breasts, go to bed to get some rest and get your partner to do the late-night feed.

Days 4–6

---

7 a.m.   Breastfeed, express from both breasts.

10 a.m.   Breastfeed.

4 p.m.   Breastfeed, express from both breasts.

10 p.m.   Express from both breasts, go to bed to get some rest and get your partner to do the late-night feed.

From day seven, you might want to continue to express at 7 a.m. when your milk supply is highest. You can use the milk to enable your partner to do the late-night feed or store it for use when your baby goes through a growth spurt.

Vary the above according to how much milk you are producing. If you are producing a reasonable amount, do your normal breastfeed and then express from both breasts, taking off the excess from the side you fed on and expressing for fifteen minutes from the other side. If you are only producing a small amount of milk, breastfeed for fifteen minutes from each side and then express for fifteen minutes from each side.

(These timings assume you are using an electric pump. Manual pumps take longer. If you're using a manual pump limit your pumping sessions to twenty-five minutes at a time or you may get sore nipples.)

Don't worry if you don't see much milk when you start expressing. It takes about two or three days for your body to respond to what you are asking it to do. The key is to keep stimulating the breasts and to stick to the plan until you see results – which you will.

My six-week-old baby doesn't go to sleep for ages after her first morning feed. She rarely sleeps before 9.30 a.m. Should I then wake her at 10 a.m. as the routine suggests or leave her to sleep longer?

At around four to six weeks some babies start staying awake longer in the morning and don't want to nap again as soon as they did before. It would be best to wake her for her next feed, but remember that you can vary this by fifteen minutes without the routine slipping. She will probably sleep a little longer during her next nap. You may soon find that she doesn't need this early nap at all.

My six-week-old baby is waking earlier at night for a feed. Could he be hungry and not getting enough milk during the day?

Babies go through a growth spurt at about six weeks. This can sometimes cause them to wake earlier at night through hunger. They need to take more milk during the day. Give your baby an extra ounce of milk or an extra five minutes on the breast during each of his daytime feeds.

'Karen's baby girl, Isabella, was four weeks old and Karen had been trying to follow my routine for settling her to sleep at night. But Isabella refused to settle at 7 p.m. and wouldn't fall asleep until around midnight. Karen and her husband were exhausted.

'I looked at the sleep log Karen had been keeping and noticed that Isabella was sleeping a lot during the day. She was also sleeping from 5.30 to 6.45 p.m., after which she had her bath, milk and was put to bed.

'The first thing we changed was her late-afternoon sleep: Karen started to wake her at 6 to 6.15 p.m. She would then have play time, nappy-off time and finally her bedtime ritual, winding down to bed.

'Karen also started to wake Isabella earlier before her feeds during the day, at least fifteen minutes, and to keep her awake after the feed for a short play time. Karen found this really hard because Isabella was very sleepy and Karen felt she was being cruel if she woke her. But she soon realized that she needed to sleep less during the day, and in particular that she needed to be awake for a while after every feed so she would break the connection between feeding and sleeping.

'It took only four days for things to slot into place and for Isabella to stay awake of her own accord after each feed. She also slept happily from 7 to 11 p.m. every evening, giving Karen a chance to catch up on her own sleep.'

Jo

Six weeks onwards . . .

What if . . .

My seven-week-old baby is really tired well before his nap times. After his mid-morning feed at 10.30 I find it really hard to play

*with him as he gets cranky. Should I wait to put him down to sleep
until 11.45 as your routine suggests or can he sleep sooner?*
It sounds as if your baby may not have slept much after his
early-morning feed and is now rather sleepy. Try to play with
him for fifteen minutes if you can, but put him down for a nap
earlier if you think he really needs it. Make sure that after the
next feed you make up for this with a slightly longer play time.

A sleep log will help you to see your baby's natural pattern of
naps and you'll be able to work out when to put him down before
he gets overtired. It will also help you develop a daytime nap
schedule that suits his own particular needs.

*My eight-week-old baby is breastfed but is given one bottle feed of
expressed milk late at night when she plays with the teat and
doesn't drink much.*
Babies who are mainly breastfed sometimes find the silicone teats
on bottles to their dislike. Try a latex teat, the sort which is usually
used for premature babies and newborns and which resembles the
breast more closely. See if she takes to it.

*My ten-week-old baby has been fed only on the breast. I now need
to offer him a bottle (of expressed breastmilk) but every time I do
so he screams and screams. I persist for about twenty minutes but
he still screams and in the end I have to give him a breastfeed.*
Many mums find that if they haven't given their baby a bottle in
the first few weeks they encounter this sort of problem further
down the line and it can be very distressing for both them and
their baby.

Your baby may be associating the bottle with hunger as you
are offering it to him for quite some time, during which he is
probably desperate for food. Try offering it for no more than a
couple of minutes before offering him the breast so that he breaks
the association with his hunger and he should begin to accept it.

'*Ten weeks after Chloe was born I wanted to go to an exercise class to try to get back in shape. It started at 7 p.m. so my partner offered to put her to bed. We were in for a surprise!*

'*As I had been breastfeeding exclusively, I made up a bottle of expressed milk, but Chloe started to scream the minute she was offered it. She would scream for twenty minutes after which I put her on the breast. It was really upsetting for all of us.*

'*Jo suggested offering the bottle a few times a day but she told me to take it away as soon as the baby started to cry and give her the breast instead. This was to stop her associating the bottle with feeling upset and hungry. It took five days of doing this to get the bottle into her mouth – but then she refused to suck. So Jo suggested getting latex teats, walking round with her while feeding, making sure she was hungry at each feed and not giving up! Four days later she finally drank a full bottle. And I made it to my exercise class.*'

Anna

My two-month-old baby is crying even though it's nowhere near his feed time – what do I do between now and then?

This is something you can encounter at any stage during your baby's first months.

It may not be hunger that is making your baby cry (see chapter 5). Go through the checklist, and if you're sure it is hunger, you can distract him until you're closer to his feed time. Play with him, put him in his rocker chair in front of the window (or even the washing machine!), play some music, give him a cuddle or pop him in a baby carrier and walk round the house, or use a dummy. A change of scenery always works wonders so you could take him for a walk in the carrier or buggy.

Don't push yourself or your baby to the point where you're both unhappy: if you feel you need to feed him before his feed time, then do. Remember – routines are meant to be flexible and the guide times can be varied by fifteen minutes either way with ease.

If he hasn't slept since his last feed, he is probably overtired and needs to sleep or he will be too tired to take a full feed when the time comes. He may even fall asleep during the feed and you will find it very hard to wake him to get him to finish his milk. Try to put him down for naps before he gets too tired. A sleep log will help you with this: keep one for at least a week and note the times that he starts to get cranky. You should see a pattern emerge, enabling you to catch his need for sleep in time.

He may be so tired that he cannot fall asleep. Help him with a dummy, or rock him in his rocker chair or pushchair, but stop the rocking before he actually falls asleep (see p. 67). Limit the use of these methods to the times he is overtired. Now that he is two months old it is important for him to learn to fall asleep without help.

My two-month-old baby throws up his feed.
Most babies have a small posset after a feed. Your baby has probably brought up less than you fear. If you pour an ounce of milk over a work surface, you'll get an idea of how much or how little your baby is actually bringing up. He may simply be getting rid of any excess milk he can't digest. If you are worried, give him an ounce or two of cooled boiled water so he doesn't get dehydrated. This should also help to settle his tummy. You may have to bring his next feed time forward by half an hour or so if he subsequently gets hungry.

If he's throwing up a lot, and does so for more than a couple of days, seek medical advice (see also chapter 11).

I give my two-month-old baby a reduced feed when she wakes in the late afternoon as you suggest in routine 4, but it doesn't seem to be enough for her and she gets really upset. Should I just give her a full feed?

A reduced feed is useful when your baby is working towards having fewer feeds every twenty-four hours (see Routines 4–7), and is designed to fill the gap that inevitably arises in the late afternoon. It's too long for your baby to last without getting hungry and fretful during her bath, but too short to fit in a full feed (which could mean she won't take a full feed before going to bed).

The best time to do this is between 5.30 and 6 p.m. before her bath. Give her a couple of ounces or ten minutes on the breast. It should be only a small amount otherwise your baby may fall asleep, or be sick in the bath or during her massage. If she still seems hungry after the reduced feed your best bet is to try to distract her. Dads sometimes arrive home around this time, and that might prove the perfect distraction.

My ten-week-old baby will sleep only for forty minutes at a time during the day and then cries until I get her up.

Every time your baby wakes up go to her and try the techniques for night-time settling (spaced soothing, see p. 161). Do this for up to fifteen minutes if she doesn't settle back to sleep. After that time you can get her up. Do the same the following day. Within a few days you should find that her naps get a little longer. Once she is sleeping through the night from 11 p.m. to 7 a.m. try putting her in her cot for naps and you may find this will help her to sleep longer during the day.

'Emma was finding that her eight-week-old baby Sophie was only sleeping for forty-five minutes during her daytime naps after which she was wide awake and wouldn't resettle.

'It turned out that Sophie was napping in a very busy and noisy room with people coming in and out. We moved her to a quieter room and I got Emma to do spaced soothing when Sophie woke up. She did this for fifteen minutes.

'For the first three days Sophie wouldn't settle back to sleep, but on the fourth she woke briefly and then resettled herself. After a week she was napping for more than an hour. Over the next few weeks her daily naps became more organized and she slept for about an hour in the morning and an hour to an hour and a quarter at lunchtime, which meant Emma could have some time to catch up with chores or even have a relaxing lunch.'

Jo

My three-month-old baby seems to be hungry all day long, every couple of hours. Is this normal?

It is normal for babies to get very hungry when they're going through growth spurts. These usually take place around day six, day twelve, three weeks and six weeks and then every few weeks after that, so it could be that your baby is going through one. If you are formula-feeding, offer an extra ounce of milk at each feed for a couple of days, and, if you are breastfeeding, always offer the second breast (or an extra five minutes if you are already doing so) or give your baby a bottle of expressed milk at the end of his feed.

An alternative would be to feed him slightly more frequently during the growth spurt, reducing the time between feeds for two to three days – this will also increase your milk supply. When you revert to the times you were on previously, your baby will find there is more milk available if he wants it.

If you are bottle-feeding it's not a good idea to give your baby more than the recommended amount for his age. It may be that your baby is very 'sucky' rather than hungry so try giving him a dummy after his feed.

'Tania was finding that bottle-feeding her eleven-week-old twins was taking her more than an hour, and at times one feed would run into the next.

'We changed the teats to the next size up and introduced a cut-off point of an hour for feeds. At the end of each feed I got Tania to throw any remaining milk away so there was no temptation to give it to the babies in between feeds. Within a matter of days they were taking their feeds in around twenty to thirty minutes.

'Tania was overjoyed as it gave her some time and space during the day.'

Jo

My three-month-old baby is so tired, cranky and hungry by the time she has had her bath that she starts screaming for food before we are ready to give it to her at 7 p.m.

Once babies reach about three months they are much more active during the day and this translates into tiredness in the evenings. You could try to give her a small feed before her bath, say at around 6 p.m. Or bring her seven o'clock feed forward a little so that she gets her milk before she gets upset.

I take my three-month-old baby out a lot and he sleeps in the buggy or the car. I'm wondering if this is as good as a sleep in his cot.

It's fine for a young baby to sleep in his buggy, and what better way for you to meet friends or do some shopping, than when he's fast asleep? Knowing when your baby's naptimes are means you can plan your trips around them.

Remember the advice on p. 67 about getting your baby to fall asleep in his buggy or car seat before you leave – if you can. Otherwise he'll get used to the idea of having motion to send him to sleep and won't be able to do without it.

In the first three months or so try to let him have as many naps as he can at home, in his moses basket, rocker chair or a stationary buggy if he prefers it. Once he's about four months old and is sleeping through the night, you can introduce him to the cot for naptimes as this is where he will get his most refreshing – and best quality – sleep. This is particularly important for his long lunchtime nap which he will probably need until he is about three years old. You don't need the room to be in total darkness during daytime naps in the cot and if you are using a lullaby soother at night you don't need this during the day either.

Your baby's daily naps are really important for his health and development and naps in a quiet, dark room in a cot will always be the best naps he can have. Would you want to take a nap while moving around a brightly lit and noisy supermarket, for example? But that doesn't mean you can't get him to take some naps in the buggy or car now and then if you need him to. Just keep a balance.

My fourteen-week-old baby doesn't like being in his cot for naps.
Once your baby has been sleeping through the night for about two weeks, it's a good idea for him to start having his daytime naps in his cot. There should be no risk now that this will confuse him, because he has already learned to differentiate between day and night. He may be unsettled at first: try the techniques for night-time settling (spaced soothing, see p. 161) for a few days. Don't despair. He will soon get used to the change. You do, however, need to commit to staying at home until this works out

and he is comfortable with the new arrangement. It would be a shame if you tried for three days and then went out on the fourth, causing your baby to fall asleep in the car or pushchair just as he was learning to nap in his cot.

If you are worried about feeling restricted by your baby's regular midday nap in his cot, there is a compensation: you will have around two hours of quiet time every day to catch up with chores. Once napping in a cot is well established, you can revert to occasional naps in the car or pushchair when you need to. Again, just keep things balanced.

My four-month-old baby is still following a three-hourly routine. (I'm breastfeeding.) I am worried that I should be stretching his feeds and moving to the next routine but he seems so happy with things as they are. On top of everything he has just started to sleep through the night. Do I have to move to a different routine?
Breastfed babies sometimes need feeding a little more often than formula-fed babies. (Formula milk takes longer to digest.) It may be that your baby *needs* to be fed every three hours. If he is happy and if you are happy then there's no reason to change anything.

It's up to you to choose a routine which suits your baby and only move on when you feel he is ready; until then stick with what you're doing. It sounds as if you have got things just right, and if your baby is sleeping through the night now all your dreams have come true.

I feel I am becoming a slave to my six-month-old's schedule. My friends say I should now be able to get out and about and bring him along.
You're not becoming a slave, you're just acknowledging the importance of healthy naps for your baby. Friends who don't understand this may not realize that you're putting your baby's needs before your own. When you do want to go out, try to

distinguish between routine days and exceptional days when things don't go quite according to plan. Disrupting your baby's sleep patterns now and then will have no long-term effects. As ever, it's about getting the balance right.

General problems

What if . . .

My friend has followed a different routine and swears by it. Should I switch to hers?
It can be confusing and unsettling for your baby if you keep chopping and changing, so if a routine is working then stick with it.

I need to be more flexible in my life than the routines seem to allow.
The routines are guidelines and you can vary and adapt them, which makes them very flexible. Think of them as forming an outline to your day so that everyone – your baby, your partner and you – knows what is happening.

I want to go away for the weekend to visit my sister but I am worried about how I will keep my baby's routine going while we travel.
Have routine, will travel . . . Routines really do make travelling easier. You simply follow what you usually do at home, sticking to the timings of your baby's feeds, play time and naps as closely as you can. It may take a little bit of preparation and planning to make sure, for example, that you don't find yourself on the motorway at feed time and nowhere near a service station.

During car journeys, take a break both for a feed and for play time: walking your baby round a car park may not seem fun to you but may be fascinating to him. When you arrive at your sister's, follow the routine as you would at home and follow your baby's bedtime ritual as closely as you can too. Your baby will find the familiarity of both routine and ritual comforting in an unfamiliar place. (See 'Travel' on p. 275 for more information.)

I have to be out of the house for most of the afternoon with my baby and I know I won't be able to feed him at the time the routine says I should.
This is where a routine can really help you, because you know when your baby is going to be hungry. Simply work out the closest time that is convenient to feed him. Remember that the feed times can usually vary by fifteen minutes either way without upsetting your baby or throwing his routine off course. Remember too that if you didn't have a routine you would have no idea when he might suddenly want to be fed and chances are that it would be at the most inconvenient time possible.

My baby has been really unwell and the routine has fallen apart.
When babies are ill routines will always take a knock and you may feel a bit frustrated that all your hard work has been for nothing – but it won't have been. The things your baby learned before he was ill won't have been forgotten. Once he's better, view the next day as a fresh start: return to the routine and you should find that your baby recognizes the cues and slips back into it with a minimum of effort.

I'm worried that my milk might dry up if I feed on a routine.
Some people claim that this is a disadvantage of routines but there's no reason to assume this will happen. The most common cause of a mum's milk drying up is exhaustion, and exhaustion is more likely if you are feeding on demand round-the-clock. If at any stage you think your milk supply is dwindling, follow the tips on p. 125 for boosting it.

I've just got used to this routine and now I feel it's being thrown up in the air because we are switching to the next one.

It's easy to feel comfortable in a routine and to worry about moving on to the next one. But you should see each change as exciting: it's part of the joy of watching your baby grow. You and your baby will probably find it takes only a few days to adapt to the new routine.

7.

Sleep: the Greatest Gift

'So many parents assume that having a baby who sleeps well is the luck of the draw: they hope they will be among the lucky ones, but accept that they might not be. I hear stories of antenatal teachers telling mums-to-be to prepare themselves for months of sleep deprivation as if that's normal. And of mums thinking it's normal to spend night after night lying on cushions on the floor watching television waiting for their baby to fall asleep in the early hours.

'Well, it isn't. I've never failed to get a baby sleeping through the night. They can't all have been "naturally" good sleepers. The fact is that you can teach any baby to sleep through the night and you can do it in the first few weeks of his life: good sleepers are made, not born.

'Parents are so relieved when I tell them it can be done, but it's nothing compared to the look of joy on their faces when it finally happens. Some call me a magician but what I do isn't magic. It's straightforward and simple.

'I often return to see the babies I've worked with months or years later, and they still sleep through the night. It makes such a difference to their families: the parents have the time and energy to enjoy their kids and get to spend time with each other in the evenings. It also makes a difference to the children: babies who sleep well are always happier babies. After all sleep is essential for your baby's development. After food it is the most important thing in his life. Sleep helps babies to grow, to process what they have learned during the day, to develop vital brain functions. What greater gift could there be?

'With your help your baby can become a great sleeper. The key is to start as early as you can, and to follow my routines at the same time: the night-time techniques pick up where the daytime routines end.

'The following two chapters will show you what to do – but first you need to find out how soon your baby can sleep well and why it is so important. That is what this chapter will tell you.'

Jo

'Something extraordinary happens every night in my house at around seven o'clock. My twin boys, who by day are rampaging two-and-a-half-year-olds, settle happily into their cots, fall asleep and sleep through the night. And they have done this since they were tiny babies.

'It's extraordinary to me because before becoming a mum I heard horror stories of babies crying through the night for months, of toddlers battling bedtime with an iron will and of parents becoming increasingly frazzled. I truly dreaded that this might happen to me but had no idea what to do about it.

'Thank goodness I met Jo. She promised that my boys would be sleeping through the night by the age of three to four months. In the early sleepless weeks it was hard at times to believe and I wondered whether she was spinning me a yarn. But Jo told me to be patient. And she was absolutely right. We got there.

'Friends couldn't believe it. Even now they are amazed

that the boys still sleep so well. It just goes to show that parenthood doesn't have to go hand-in-hand with sleep deprivation.

'I promise that you can get there too, that you will be as thrilled as I was when your babies sleep through the night, and that you will still be smiling months – and years – later on.

'Having sleeping babies transformed all our lives. We thrived on being well-rested parents: much as we loved the boys we needed time to ourselves in the evenings. And the boys seemed so much happier once they were sleeping well. I feel I've given them a special gift – a gift we have all been able to enjoy.

'That gift is now within your reach too.'
Barbara

The 'long stretch' of sleep

Parents sometimes assume that babies are naturally either good or bad sleepers and that there is little they can do about this. It comes as a huge surprise to most people to learn that all healthy full-term babies are capable of sleeping through the night by four months, if not sooner. All they need to get there is a helping hand.

By the age of six weeks every baby has the capacity to sleep one continuous long stretch of four to six hours in every twenty-four-hour period. Ideally this should be in the middle of the night. (The long stretch is sometimes referred to as the 'core night'.) It may not sound much, but it is the beginning of good night-time sleeping patterns.

By the age of seven to nine weeks that long stretch of sleep can extend to seven or eight hours, and by the age of three months to eleven or even twelve – a full night's sleep, which every baby

can achieve by four months. And if you think four months is a
long time to wait, rest assured that many babies get there sooner.

Your baby's weight is another useful guide as to when he
should start to sleep well: many babies seem able to sleep a long
stretch of up to about eight hours when they reach about 12lb in
weight, and a full night – twelve hours – when they reach about
15 or 16lb.

The following chart is a guide to what babies are capable of.

Baby's age/weight	Number of hours (approx.) he is capable of sleeping without waking for a feed
6 weeks	4 to 6 hours
7–9 weeks (or 12lb)	7 to 8 hours
9–12 weeks	8 to 11 hours
3–4 months (or 15–16lb)	12 hours
6 months	If you are still giving your baby night feeds at this age, you may be interfering with his sleep.*

This chart applies to healthy term babies. If your baby is premature you will have to adjust the ages for his prematurity. If
your baby has colic these times may take longer to achieve (see
chapter 11). Serious illnesses can also set a baby back.

Remember that the chart shows only a baby's *potential*. Most
babies will need help to realize that potential, which is where the
secrets of sleep outlined in the next chapter come in. And, of
course, every child is an individual, and some will learn more

* Richard Ferber, author of *Solve Your Child's Sleep Problems*, warns that
night-feeding when no longer necessary may affect a child's body rhythms
and interfere with a good night's sleep.

quickly than others. A small number of babies will even do it without help, but leaving something as important as this to chance is a high-risk strategy.

Your aim is to get your baby to sleep these long stretches as soon as he can.

Why it's good for babies to sleep well

> 'I thought getting a baby to sleep was for the parents' benefit, but I've changed my thinking: it's fundamental for the baby. Hannah was so much happier once she started to sleep well.'
> **Ruth**

What are the benefits of getting your baby to sleep well as soon as possible?

First, once you start getting some sleep, everyone will benefit, because a rested parent is always better than a tired one.

Secondly, babies who learn to sleep well at an early age continue to sleep well – bringing everyone many years of night-time peace. Equally, babies who do not can carry sleep problems into toddlerhood and beyond.

Thirdly, it seems that an unbroken night's sleep may be more important for your baby's development than you realize. Good sleeping patterns may make for happier and even brighter babies, according to research.

In his book *Healthy Sleep Habits, Happy Child*, Dr Marc Weissbluth, director of the Sleep Disorder Center at the Children's Memorial Hospital in Chicago, makes a powerful case for the link between healthy sleep patterns and the healthy development of a baby's brain. Dr Weissbluth conducted a study of sixty babies at five months old and found that the babies who slept longer were happy, easy-going and had longer attention spans than those who didn't. The poor sleepers by contrast were irritable and fussy. Babies who are more alert and able to concentrate, claims Dr Weissbluth, are also able to learn better; hence the link between sleep and intelligence. His view is supported by other research on older children that shows that those who sleep well also do better at school. Yes, good sleepers may grow up to be clever. What more powerful case could there be for helping your baby to get it right?

It may be easier to understand the effect that poor sleep has on a baby's ability to learn if we think about the effect that a bad night has on us. We all feel the same after broken sleep: we either wake at the usual time in the morning and are exhausted for the rest of the day, or we lie in, and find we can't get to sleep the following night. If things go badly, this can become a vicious circle.

Some of us resort to a catnap during the day, but this is a mixed blessing if we wake up feeling worse than we did before. That's because the whole pattern of our day has been disturbed. Under these circumstances, none of us functions at our best. How often have we had to apologize to friends or colleagues for being too tired to think clearly because we've had a bad night's sleep? How often do we complain that we are ill when in fact we are simply tired and run down?

It is no different for a baby. Without a full stretch of uninterrupted sleep at night and good-quality naps during the day, he will not be at his best. He may be cranky, fussy, or miserable. He may become so overtired that he finds it difficult to fall asleep at all, and ends up so exhausted that he sleeps all day and cannot sleep the following night either.

His alertness during the day depends on how well he sleeps. If he is not fully alert his concentration will be poor, his attention span will be shorter, he will be easily distracted and, the argument goes, he won't be able to learn as well from his environment.

Nor is long-term cumulative sleep deprivation different for

your baby from what it is for you. It can take a terrible toll on your health and well-being. And if you are not sleeping because your baby is not sleeping, you will be sleep-deprived too.

Many parents notice how much happier their babies seem to be once they sleep well. And this is likely to make parents happier too.

Why babies need help to sleep well

Here is a last word from Dr Weissbluth. 'It comes as a surprise to many parents that healthy sleep habits do *not* develop automatically . . . the process of falling asleep and staying asleep is learned behaviour.'

The good news is that teaching your baby to sleep well is easy. But as with so many things, it is easier to instil good sleep habits from the start than it is to correct bad sleep habits later. You can begin from the very day you bring your baby home from hospital. But if you cannot start straightaway, for whatever reason, don't despair. It is never too late. The seven secrets of sleep will be your guide.

Remember

- Babies who sleep well are happier and may even become brighter children
- Poor sleeping patterns will not help your baby and may even affect his development
- Good sleep habits can last into toddlerhood and beyond
- Sleep problems can persist into toddlerhood and beyond
- It's never too early to teach your baby to sleep well
- A rested parent is a better parent.

8.

The Seven Secrets of Sleep

'I once met a mum who found that her little baby slept very happily . . . if he was lying on his mum's tummy. So she let him do so, and within a few days it was the *only* place he would sleep . . . Before long she was absolutely exhausted because, although her baby slept well, she didn't sleep a wink.

'Parents are sometimes puzzled when I say I can "teach" their baby to sleep well. They can't believe that small babies are ready to learn. But from the day he is born your baby is like a sponge, absorbing information and learning from his environment. He also learns from you, both from what you *do* (including helping him to sleep) and from what you *don't do*.

'Rocking a baby to sleep, letting him fall asleep on the breast or bottle, rushing to his side every time he wakes or putting him on your tummy — any or all of these may help him get to sleep. But he may then decide that's the only way he can do so.

'What I do instead is to show parents how to teach their babies to fall asleep on their own. They need this skill so that when they wake during the night (which they will continue to do) they don't need help to settle again. You may be surprised to hear that even babies who "sleep through the night" wake up several times. (In fact we all do.) Those babies who "sleep through" simply go back to sleep without help.

'My technique for doing this is called "spaced soothing"

and it is gentle, caring and fabulously effective. You can easily use it too.

'I firmly believe that you can – and should – start to teach your baby to sleep well from the day he arrives home, or as soon after as you can manage. I have worked with enough babies to know that they start learning from the minute they are born and very quickly understand what is expected of them. It is so much easier if you do this from the start, otherwise your baby may pick up bad habits which will have to be unlearned, and you may be too exhausted to see it through.

'My other task is to get parents to stretch, and then drop, their baby's night-time feeds so their baby will give up wanting milk in the night as soon as he is able to, so a full night's sleep can happen sooner rather than later.

'You can start stretching your baby's sleep once he is about two weeks old (assuming he was born at term and is healthy – you must wait for a premature baby to reach 7lb). Again, you can leave it until later, but it will be harder to achieve.

'This chapter will tell you about the seven secrets of sleep, which are key to getting a baby to sleep through the night.

'(By the way – it only took a couple of days to wean the "tummy-sleeper" off his mum's tummy and to get him to sleep happily in his own cot. His mum jokes that if I hadn't shown her what to do he would still be sleeping on her tummy now – at the age of two.)'

Jo

'Can you really teach a newborn baby something? I believe you can, and that teaching a baby to sleep well is one of the kindest things you can do. To teach is to love.'

Barbara

The seven secrets of sleep

The first secret . . .

is to start every night with a *bedtime ritual.* Babies and toddlers relish routine and ritual. They like to know what is coming next. They like certainty. It doesn't matter what that ritual is as long as you follow it consistently every night, and the last stages should always take place in your baby's bedroom. This will help him learn to love being in his room and never to feel it is a place to which he is sent to be on his own. And if you keep the ritual the same night after night, he will thrive on it and actively *enjoy* going to bed.

You can start a bedtime ritual whenever you feel ready – from as early as day one. But if you do not feel organized or confident that early on, try to make a start as soon afterwards as you can. The ritual can be followed for months, if not years afterwards (with modifications as your baby gets older, of course). It's easy and fun. And if you want to adapt it in ways that suit you, that's fine as long as you are consistent night after night.

The second secret . . .

of night-time sleep is to *treat every hour between 7 p.m. and 7 a.m. as night-time* and *never* to deviate from that. You can, and ideally should, start to do this as soon as your baby arrives home (but again, it is never too late to start, so don't give up).

Your baby will soon understand what daytime is like. It is busy and exciting, with games and activities, cuddles and 'conversations' with mum or dad. Every day there are new and interesting things to see.

For a baby to learn that night-time is different, it has to be different. At night it should be dark and quiet with no talking, no cuddles (unless, of course, you need to comfort an unhappy baby), no eye contact (if you can manage it), and certainly no games or activities. In short, it should be so unexciting that your baby will soon learn that it's not worth trying to stay awake.

Ideally your baby should spend all the night hours in his bedroom and, even if he is unsettled, it is best not to take him out. Given the opportunity once, he will want to come out time and again, which will not help to settle him. Indeed it will probably wake him more. (The only exception to this rule, naturally, is if your baby is unwell.)

This applies even in the last couple of hours before the day starts when it can be tempting to allow a baby to get up because he is wide awake. The risk is that he will then assume that when you get him up it is daytime and, logically, that daytime starts at that time every day.

Blackout blinds or very dark curtains are a great help here, particularly in the summer months (see p. 13).

The third secret . . .
is *never to let your baby fall asleep in your arms or while he is feeding.*

Always put your baby down *awake* – whether at night in his cot or during the day in his moses basket or rocker chair – or he will not learn to settle to sleep on his own. Try to do this from the day your baby is born or as soon afterwards as you can.

Think about your own sleep habits and you can see why this matters so much. Imagine you are in the habit of falling asleep with the radio playing softly in the background. Every time you wake up you need the radio to help you fall asleep again. One night you find the radio is broken. Can you fall asleep without it? Only with great difficulty.

Now imagine that your radio is the equivalent, for your baby, of being held in your arms, or of the comfort of a breast or bottle to suck on. He will very soon come to rely on it in the same way that you rely on your radio. Take it away from him one night and he won't be able to fall asleep without it.

When he wakes during the night he will also want you to help him return to his slumbers. (All babies wake several times a night.) It is tempting to rock him to sleep in your arms, not least because it allows you to return to the comfort of your bed more quickly, but the more often you give in to this temptation, the harder it will be to break this pattern. Some parents still rock their one-year-olds to sleep because it is a habit they have got into and find hard to break, so it really is worth trying to avoid this.

The fourth secret . . .

is a technique called '*spaced soothing*'. You can use this whenever your baby is unsettled. It will help to calm him and prepare him to fall asleep on his own. It's the key to the whole process.

Spaced soothing is wonderful because it means you can calm your baby and reassure him that you are there for him without always picking him up – which can make him more wakeful and become a pattern of behaviour that he wants you to repeat. The other great joy is that, although it is effective at helping a baby to fall asleep of his own accord, it never requires you to leave your baby to cry for long periods. As a tool, its main use is at night, although there may be times during the day when you can use it to help your baby to nap. It is explained fully in the next chapter.

The fifth secret . . .

is *not to rush to your baby at every sound but to go to him only when he needs you*. Rushing to him too soon can actively prevent him from sleeping.

Babies make many noises while they are falling asleep, while they are asleep, while they drift in and out of sleep, and in between phases of light and deep sleep. Newborns have more light sleep than adults and make all manner of noises during it. Many of these squawks, grizzles and whimpers are a natural part of a baby's sleep or his attempts to drop off to sleep: some babies need to let off energy by crying in order to get to sleep. They don't need mum or dad at their side all the time getting in the way.

Think of it from your baby's point of view. He is drifting off to sleep, grumbling as he unwinds, trying to settle himself and find a comfortable position. Suddenly, just as he's about to nod off, the process is interrupted. Imagine how infuriating it must be. But repeat this often enough, and he may never learn to fall asleep because he is repeatedly being dragged back from the brink by an over-solicitous mum or dad.

How frustrated would you be if every time you made a sound, twitched or sighed as you drifted off to sleep, your partner elbowed you and woke you up to check you're OK? Would you not rather be left in peace?

This does not mean that you will ignore your baby during the night, but you will go to him only when you are sure he really needs you. Parents sometimes feel they're being cruel if they don't respond to their baby's every sound. If this worries you remember that no baby ever grew up feeling unloved or suffering psychological damage through learning how to settle himself to sleep.

The sixth secret . . .
is to give your baby a late-night feed, or '*dream feed*', at the same time every night (until, of course, he no longer needs it because he is sleeping through). A good time to give him this feed is at 11 p.m. *whether he is already awake or not*. Often he won't be, so you will need to wake him.

The idea is not only to make sure that your baby has a full tummy as he enters the small hours (although that helps). It is also a way of delaying the onset of his long stretch of sleep (see previous chapter) when it starts to happen, so that it takes place in the middle of the night when you too can get some sleep. If you wait until later to feed your baby (when he wakes naturally), he will have had his long stretch of sleep already and it will have happened too early.

The dream feed gets its name from the fact that babies are very sleepy at this time of night, so much so that some almost sleep all the way through it.

You can start an 11 p.m. dream feed from the age of about two weeks. Until then many babies will wake earlier and you should feed them then. Once they reach two weeks they will either start to sleep through until 11 p.m. or you can stretch the feed (see below) by fifteen minutes every three days until you reach eleven o'clock.

The dream feed is the last of the night-time feeds to be dropped. That happens once a baby is sleeping from 11 p.m. to 7 a.m., somewhere around the age of three to four months.

The seventh secret . . .
is to establish a *base time* for when you feed your baby in the middle of the night and never to feed him any earlier.

The base time is when your baby needs to be fed. Feed him too early, when he doesn't need feeding, and you run the risk that a long stretch of sleep will never happen, let alone lengthen. Your baby may also get so used to being fed at that early time that he will set his internal 'alarm clock' to wake every night accordingly in expectation of a feed (and, of course, the bonus of time spent with mum or dad).

By waiting until your baby needs to be fed you are encouraging him to sleep as long as he is able. You should manage to work out what your baby's base time is by the time he is two to three weeks old. Once you have established a base time you can start to stretch it, which you can do with the help of spaced soothing. You will stretch it bit by bit until eventually the night-time feed disappears and you have reached your goal: a baby who sleeps through the night.

Seven secrets to sleeping through the night

1. *Follow a bedtime ritual* consistently every night.

2. *Treat every hour between 7 p.m. and 7 a.m. as night-time.*

3. Never let your baby fall asleep in your arms or while he is feeding: *always lay your baby down awake.*

4. *Use spaced soothing to calm and settle him* so he can learn to fall asleep by himself.

5. *Don't rush in at every sound* but remember the fact that many of the noises a baby makes are his attempts to fall asleep and you may disrupt him.

6. *Give your baby a dream feed* at around 11 p.m. – until he is ready to sleep through the night.

7. *Set a base time for his middle-of-the-night feed and never feed him before it*: stretch that time gradually until your baby sleeps through the night.

What will help me to follow these secrets?

First, it is important to realize that getting a baby to sleep through the night is easier with a baby fed on a routine. This is because routine-fed babies are more likely to drink all the milk they need during the day and to be less hungry at night than those who are demand-fed. They are also less likely to wake as they have no expectations of frequent feeds.

Secondly, it is a good idea to make sure you and your partner have agreed in advance to follow the secrets of sleep and the techniques they require, to avoid middle-of-the-night confusion.

If you get very tired it might help to take turns on the night-shift, or to split the hours of darkness between you.

Thirdly, you need to use the techniques every night. Following them one day, but not the next, will leave your baby confused. Consistency is the key.

Fourthly, please don't view them as a quick fix; there are no quick fixes with babies. At times you may feel that progress is slow, but have faith in your baby and don't let him down by giving up too soon. You *will* get there, together.

Do formula-fed babies sleep through the night earlier than breastfed babies?

This is a hot topic among new mums . . . It may be that those breastfed babies who do take longer to sleep through the night do so not because of the breastmilk itself, but because breastfeeding mums may be more likely to use breastfeeding as a way of comforting a baby or sending him off to sleep. This becomes a habit and the baby does not learn to fall asleep on his own. A study indicating that breastfed babies can sleep through the night as soon as formula-fed babies if they are fed on a routine is reported by Gary Ezzo and Robert Bucknam, authors of *On Becoming Babywise*.

> 'I am often asked whether formula-fed babies sleep through the night sooner than breastfed babies. Many people assume they do – but I don't think you can generalize that easily: I know many babies fed solely on breastmilk who slept through the night at an early age. The key, I believe, is the *way* a baby is fed, i.e. routine. Breastmilk or formula doesn't make a huge difference.
>
> 'You might like to know that many (but not all) babies

I work with, from around four to six weeks of age, *do* sleep slightly longer if given formula for the dream feed. If mums choose to do this, it's usually so that they can leave this feed to their partner, and catch up on sleep before the middle-of-the-night feed. You may worry that this is a slippery slope towards giving up breastfeeding altogether, but I promise you that it isn't. The main reason mums give up breastfeeding is exhaustion; anything that buys you extra sleep will be worth its weight in gold – and help to preserve your strength for producing breastmilk.'
Jo

What are the milestones to sleeping through the night?

There are four stages to reaching the goal of twelve hours of uninterrupted sleep. Each one is an important milestone, and when you reach it you should feel justifiably proud. Assuming you follow the secrets of sleep from soon after your baby is born, this is what you can expect:

1. You can hope to see results just one to two weeks after your baby is born, by getting him to settle easily after his 7 p.m. feed and to sleep until the late-night dream feed at 11 p.m. This is a sign that your baby is already learning good sleeping patterns.

2. The next milestone comes when your baby (with your help) achieves his long stretch of four to six hours of sleep, after the dream feed. This can happen once your baby is around six weeks old. This demonstrates that your baby's sleep patterns are falling into place and he is sleeping his long stretch at the right time of the night.

3. The third milestone is when your baby sleeps from the dream feed until 7 a.m. the next morning. This will feel like a real breakthrough, not least because your own sleep patterns will now be returning to normal. You can hope to achieve this target any time after your baby has reached around ten weeks old.

4. Now your goal is in sight: the fourth and final milestone, when you drop the dream feed and your baby sleeps from around 7 p.m. until seven the following morning. It can happen when a baby is as young as twelve weeks old, although, once again, some are bound to take a little longer. (Anecdotally boys seem to be a week or two behind girls.)

Will your baby now sleep 'like a baby' for ever? No, he won't. There will be times, particularly if he is ill or unsettled, when he will have periods of wakefulness and he will need your help to soothe him. But the foundations you and he have built should mean that disruptions are temporary. When they pass, your baby will revert quickly to what he has learned – sleeping through the night. The next chapter will show you how to make this happen.

Stages to go through for night-time sleep

1. Settling after the 7 p.m. feed	This can take as little as a week and two weeks at the most.
2. Sleeping a long stretch after the dream feed	A baby is capable of sleeping a long stretch by the age of six weeks (see chart on p. 142). (If you start the techniques after your baby reaches six weeks, it will take you about two weeks to get your baby sleeping this long. It will be a little harder than it would have been if you had started earlier, but it certainly can be done.)
3. Sleeping from the dream feed to the next morning	This can be achieved from around ten weeks. (If your baby is older than ten weeks when you start the techniques, it will take you about two weeks to get here.)
4. Dropping the dream feed and sleeping through the night	Around twelve to sixteen weeks. (If you start the techniques after your baby has reached this age, it will take you about two weeks to achieve. It will be quite hard by this age but still possible. If you leave it until after your baby has reached six months it will be very hard indeed.)

9.

How to Get Your Baby Sleeping Through the Night

'Feeding a baby in the middle of the night was never my idea of fun. I have heard mothers describing night-feeding as a wonderful, private time for them and their baby, but for me it was gruelling . . . There were times I was so tired I felt like weeping.

'So one of my priorities was getting the boys to sleep through the night as soon as possible. But I knew so many people with babies who didn't sleep that I did wonder whether it could be done.

'Jo showed me that it was not only possible but straightforward. Anyone can teach their baby to sleep through the night with a few simple but effective techniques. All you need is a bit of commitment.

'I know that while you are working at it, it can be tough going. My plea to you is to have faith: the rewards are enormous, both for you and your baby. This chapter will show you what to do, starting at the moment you finish your daytime routine. Believe me: it really does work.'
Barbara

You start with *Secret 1: the bedtime ritual.* To get your baby in the mood for night-time you should give him a bath, although in the early weeks you might prefer just to top 'n' tail him (see p. 34).

After the bath take your baby into his bedroom, lay him on his changing mat and put his nappy on. Once he is about four weeks old, you can give him a gentle massage using aqueous cream, baby massage oil or grapeseed oil (see baby massage on page 36). You could play some soothing music and this will soon become a cue to your baby to wind down; you might find this music continues to be a cue for months if not years.

Most babies love being massaged but if yours reacts by crying (which some do) wait a few days and try again. It is worth persevering because it can become a key component of your baby's bedtime ritual and one of the best parts of the day. Babies can be massaged until they are several months old and when they start to wriggle at every opportunity – after which it is nearly impossible.

Now you need to start following *Secret 2: treat every hour between now and 7 a.m. as night-time*. Make sure the curtains are drawn and/or the blackout blind is down. Some parents balk at the idea of blackout blinds but they really do help your baby to understand the difference between night and day.

Dress your baby in his night clothes (don't forget to place them within easy reach beforehand), lower the lights and give him his feed. Try not to talk to him now. You are trying to send a clear message that the day is over and it is time to wind down. Calm him if he needs it with a gentle sssshhhhhh sound, which is similar to the sounds inside the womb and will reassure him. When he has finished feeding, wind him. You may have to spend about ten minutes doing this; any wind left will make it hard for him to settle.

Now you can swaddle him (see p. 62 for a discussion on swaddling), switch off any music you have been playing and *lay him in his cot awake – Secret 3*. If you have a Slumber Bear or a lullaby soother switch it on, turn off the lights, say goodnight (with conviction) and leave the room, either closing the door behind you or pulling it to. Some parents don't like closing the door on their baby, but if you leave it ajar make sure no light spills into the room from outside.

It may seem daft to say goodnight to a baby, but remember he is already watching, listening and learning, even if he does not understand the meaning of the words. Repeating them every evening will ensure he soon learns to associate them with the beginning of his night.

Parents sometimes get night lights for their babies, fearing they may be frightened by the dark. There is no need to worry. Your newborn baby spent nine months in darkness in the womb where he felt secure so the dark is his greatest friend, making him feel he is in a wonderfully safe place. A night light or a baby light projector will only distract him.

The bedtime ritual

1. Bath/Top 'n' tail
2. Nappy
3. Massage
4. Dress
5. Lights low
6. Feed
7. Wind
8. Swaddle
9. Bed
10. Lights out
11. Say goodnight
12. Leave.

What happens next?

If, after you have put your baby to bed, he is still unsettled, the first thing you should always do is *wait*. Most babies cry out briefly before settling themselves. This is their way of unwinding and is completely normal. Rushing to your baby during these first few moments will interrupt the process of getting off to sleep.

If your baby is still unsettled after a couple of minutes, go to him, keeping the lights as low as possible, and try to work out why he's crying (see chapter 5). The most likely reasons – particularly for a baby in the first four weeks of life – are wind or hunger. Pick him up, still swaddled, and check for a burp. Check for hunger: he may be rooting or butting his head against your shoulder. Or you can put your (clean) finger against his lips to see if he grabs it immediately with his mouth. These are reliable and simple checks for babies up to around six weeks and useful while you are still getting to know your baby and trying to work out when he has had a full feed. Once your baby is older and you know him better, you will find it easier to gauge when he is satisfied. If he seems to be hungry, give him some more milk, then settle him again exactly as above.

He may now settle, but if he doesn't, *Secret 4: spaced soothing* comes into play. This is your helper from the moment you put your baby in his cot after his evening feed to the minute he gets up the next morning.

Spaced soothing is a way of calming an unsettled baby and enabling him to fall asleep on his own. It imposes a very short time limit on any crying. You can't hope to teach a baby to get himself to sleep without some crying, but it doesn't have to feel at all uncomfortable. Babies need to be given the opportunity to cry for a while as it can help them to fall asleep. Going to a baby as soon as he cries can take away the opportunity. The spaced soothing technique is based on the principle that you never let your baby cry for more than a few minutes because he needs to feel confident that you are always there for him. This is how it works.

At night, whenever your baby is unsettled, first listen to the sound of his cry. Is he distressed or is he simply trying to unwind? A baby who is simply grizzling does not need comforting. It is his way of settling, of releasing tension. Don't deny him this. Remember *Secret 5: don't rush in at every sound.*

If this is your first baby you may be baffled by the idea

that you can distinguish between the different sounds he makes, between grizzles and cries, but it shouldn't take long for you to work it out. A continuous scream is a genuine cry. A grizzle stops and starts or may even be a faint-sounding whimper. These are all signs of a baby who wants to sleep but is simply fretting as he tries to do so.

If you are sure the cry is one of distress, you should *wait for about one minute* from when he started to cry. Any sooner and you are not giving your baby the chance to calm himself and fall asleep. Any sooner and he may also work out how to have you as a permanent companion at his bedside. When the minute is up, go to him, but keep the lights low and don't pick him up.

Now try the following soothing techniques to calm him:

- Whisper 'ssshhhhhhhhh' repeatedly, very softly.
- Using your index finger stroke your baby at his soothing point (sometimes known as the 'third eye') in the middle of his forehead just above the eyebrows, down between the eyes towards the bridge of the nose. Most babies quieten instantly when you do this. You could also try stroking his temple.
- Place the palm of your hand on your baby's chest to make him feel secure.
- If you are using a Slumber Bear or lullaby soother switch it on.
- As a very last resort, give him a dummy, but remove it before he falls into a deep sleep.

As soon as you hear your baby's cry soften, weaken or turn into a grizzle, leave him. It is really important to leave at this point even though you may be tempted to stay a little longer to ensure that he does fall asleep. The temptation is great – not just to ensure that he really has dropped off, but also to save yourself a trip if he wakes again soon after. But the only way you can give him the opportunity to fall asleep on his own, and the confidence that he can do it without your help, is by leaving him. If he is sleeping in your room, move away and out of sight of the cot. If he is in his own room leave the room.

Using the soothing techniques should calm a baby within about two minutes. If you find that it is persistently taking longer, or indeed that he cannot be soothed, there may be a reason: you should check the list of minor ailments in chapter 11.

If, after you leave, your baby starts crying again, wait until you are sure it is a cry, wait for a minute as you did before, then add one more minute before going to him and soothing him. Repeat this as often as you need to, adding about a minute each time, but never wait longer than around five minutes in total. If you find that five minutes of crying is too long to bear, just reduce the time. The key is to soothe him and leave as soon as he calms down, giving him the opportunity to fall asleep on his own.

If at any stage your baby gets upset and can't be soothed, you can pick him up and give him a cuddle. This is particularly important for babies under about four weeks old. They cannot calm themselves so you will need to do more cuddling during your spaced soothing than you will with a baby who is older.

There is nothing wrong with cuddling or rocking your baby if you feel it is what he needs and what you want to do. But try to make it your last, rather than your first response and remember Secret 3: never let him fall asleep in your arms. Put your baby down immediately his cry softens, soothe him and leave. (You may find that picking up your baby makes him more agitated and is counterproductive, in which case stick to the soothing techniques.)

You can vary the spacing of your visits if you feel you need to. For example, if you are waiting for four minutes but your baby is getting unhappy well before the four minutes are up, you can go to him sooner in order to soothe him before he gets too upset. The key is to repeat the action time and again, always leaving your baby when he is calm, until eventually he falls asleep on his own.

Spaced soothing

- Wait until you are sure your baby is crying and not just grizzling or unwinding.
- Wait about a minute.
- Go to his cot, keep the lights low.
- Say 'ssshhhhhhh'.
- Stroke his soothing point between the eyes gently from his forehead to the end of his nose.
- If he doesn't settle, rest the palm of your hand firmly on his chest to make him feel secure.
- Switch on his Slumber Bear or lullaby soother.
- Give him a dummy as a last, rather than a first, resort.
- Leave him as soon as you hear his crying soften – you don't have to try all the soothing techniques before leaving. You must leave his side – don't be tempted to stay and watch him fall asleep.
- If your baby is still unsettled, wait until you are sure he is crying, then wait about two minutes. Go to him and follow the steps above.
- If your baby is still unsettled, do the same, waiting about three minutes and follow the above.
- Continue until your spacing is at a maximum of about five minutes (or less if you find this too difficult).
- Keep doing this until eventually your baby falls asleep by himself.
- If at any stage your baby becomes agitated or upset, shorten the space between your visits.

- If at any stage the soothing techniques don't calm him, you can pick him up and give a cuddle to comfort him until he calms, especially with a baby under four weeks old, but don't let him fall asleep in your arms. Put him down awake as soon as he is calm.
- If you have to do this repeatedly on the first few nights don't despair: remind yourself what a great job you are doing to help your baby. If you are consistent it will get easier within a matter of days.

It may take many, many visits to your baby in the first few days before he falls asleep unaided. The process can last an hour – or even more. As you traipse back and forth it will be quite understandable if frustration sets in – or even disbelief that what you are attempting will ever work. That's when the idea of rocking your baby to sleep, or taking him out of his room, or even sitting him down beside you while you eat dinner can seem really tempting. But it really is worth resisting temptation – for your sake and his.

(Remember that if your baby is very unsettled and cannot be soothed at all, even intermittently, there may be an underlying reason: look at chapter 11 on common ailments such as colic, and if you are concerned about your baby's health you should always consult your doctor.)

If you persevere your baby will settle himself to sleep on his own after about seven days and sleep all the way to the dream feed soon after. (If you start to follow these techniques after your baby has reached six weeks it may take a few days longer.) You can be very proud that you have reached the first step on the road towards having a baby who sleeps through the night: this is a sign that the next stages are not far round the corner.

'Lydia was 7lb 10 oz and had a difficult birth resulting in an emergency caesarean. Once she was about a week old we would bath her every night at seven and then I breastfed her. She was swaddled and put in her moses basket in the darkened bedroom. The first three nights we had to go back up to her five or six times, and Jo showed me how to use spaced soothing each time, until she settled. Sometimes we realized she needed a little more milk, but more often she would only need a stroke on her nose or a dummy to calm her.

'At first she woke around 10.30 p.m., so we tried to make her wait until she reached a little nearer to 11 p.m. (spaced soothing again). After five nights of running up and down the stairs I was getting worried that this would never end, and we would never be at the table at the same time for a meal. It did seem like a very long week.

'On day six we only had to go up once and she had to be woken at 11 p.m. for her feed. It was on day eight that it all fell into place. We put her down, said goodnight, and ate our evening meal without having to go to her once. We were so relieved . . .'

Annabel

Once your baby has settled to sleep, you can wait until eleven o'clock before *Secret 6: the dream feed.* (For normal birthweight babies under two weeks old it will usually need to be a little earlier. Your baby will probably wake before 11 p.m. for a feed but try not to give it before 10.30. Once your baby reaches two weeks you can stretch this by fifteen minutes at a time to 11 p.m. – see below on how to stretch feeds.)

Luck will usually have it that at 11 p.m. your baby is fast asleep and you are dozing too. You may decide that it's crazy to wake a baby in the hope of getting him to sleep more. There is method in the madness. You and your baby are working towards getting his first long stretch of sleep, and making sure that it happens at the most convenient time of the night – when you are asleep.

By waking your baby at 11 p.m. you are preventing the long stretch from happening too early. If you don't wake him at eleven he will have his long stretch between about 8 p.m. and midnight/ 1 a.m. at which point he will wake up. You will be no more inclined to get up then than you were at 11 p.m. Worse still, your baby will now only doze until the morning as his long stretch sleep has been and gone.

So the 11 p.m. dream feed is really important. If you feel yourself wobbling, try having a nap at around 9 p.m. and take heed of this story:

> '*I found with Hadleigh that the most difficult thing was the dream feed. I simply couldn't bear to do it. I was so tired that getting up at eleven was the last thing I wanted to do. And Hadleigh was so sleepy at that time it seemed silly. I decided it was only worth doing if I saw immediate results – but I didn't. So I waited until Hadleigh woke, between midnight and 1 a.m., and I fed him then.*
>
> '*After that his sleep was very light and he would wake often. By about 5 a.m. we were both so exhausted that I would take him into bed to settle him so I could get some sleep myself. I didn't have the energy to follow the other night-time techniques and stretch his night-time feeds and we didn't manage to cut them out until he was nine months old. He was so used to interrupted nights by then that he didn't go on to sleep through a whole night until he was about a year old (and even then he would still wake some nights).*'
> **Nic**

Here are some tips regarding the dream feed.

Babies are often in a very deep sleep at this time, so to help you wake your baby, turn the lights on (low) and change his nappy. Don't be put off if his eyes are still closed. He may not open his eyes at all but he will be hungry enough to take a feed and will do so even with his eyes closed (which is why it is called 'dream feed'). It is important that you encourage him to take a full feed, even if he is sleepy. There is no need to wind him during the feed and you may find he doesn't need winding at the end: babies are so relaxed during this feed they tend not to gulp as much air as during other feeds.

If your baby wakes before 11 p.m. try spaced soothing to get him back to sleep. If he won't resettle you can feed him earlier for a few days and then stretch the feeds until he starts to sleep on until 11 p.m.

Some parents find 11 p.m. too late. You can bring it forward to 10.45 p.m. or 10.30 p.m. – any earlier and your baby may not take much milk as this feed will be too close to his previous feed. He may then wake sooner in the middle of the night.

Once they get close to sleeping through the night (from around ten weeks), some babies start to take less and less milk at this feed. If this happens, there is no need to make your baby drink more than he wants.

Once your baby has had his dream feed, settle him exactly as before. If he does not settle, do what you did at bedtime, checking first for wind or hunger and then using spaced soothing. You may have to soothe him time after time before he falls asleep: in the early days this can take an hour or more. But if you are consistent it will only be a matter of days before your baby will settle himself quickly and stay asleep until he is ready for his next feed.

So now your baby goes to sleep on his own after his 7 p.m. feed. You are waking him at 11 p.m. for his dream feed. And he is settling (reasonably) soon afterwards.

The next step is *Secret 7: set a base time for the middle-of-the-*

night feed. Never feed before that time and stretch it gradually until your baby sleeps through the night.

The base time is the time your baby needs to be fed and is easy to calculate. In the first few weeks of life most babies who have their dream feed at 11 p.m. (and settle back to sleep around 11.30–11.45), will need their next feed around three hours later, at about 2.30 a.m. If your baby wakes before 2 a.m. it is unlikely he is hungry. If he wakes after 2 a.m. but before 2.30 a.m. try to use spaced soothing either to get him to fall asleep or simply to calm him and stretch his wait until 2.30. Tempting though it may be to feed a baby who wakes earlier than 2.30 as a way for everyone to get straight back to sleep, it is not a good idea. He may not be ready for a full feed and will simply need to be fed again soon after.

Assuming your baby feeds at 2.30 a.m. this now becomes your base time. If he sleeps past that time, all the better: the later time is the base time. If you cannot stretch him past 2.15, make that your base time. When you feed him now keep the lights low, try not to talk to him and avoid eye contact. His nappy does not need changing unless it is dirty (when he sleeps through the night there will be no nappy changes). When you have fed him, settle him again exactly as before, always checking for hunger or wind at the first cry and then using spaced soothing to help him fall asleep on his own if you need to.

You should now stick to the base time and never feed your baby any earlier because you know he does not need to be fed. If he does wake earlier, used spaced soothing to help him fall asleep or keep him calm or distracted until it is time for his feed.

After a few days your baby should sleep right up until his base time without waking. Once he has slept to the base time for three days in five you can nudge the base time forward by fifteen minutes, so that the gap between feeds is stretched: this will encourage him to sleep a longer stretch. If your base time was 2.30, your new base time will be 2.45. Assuming he still wakes at 2.30, use spaced soothing to settle him back to sleep, or to keep him calm or distracted until 2.45 when you feed him.

Soon – after a few days or a week at most – your baby will sleep until 2.45. When he has done this for three nights in five you nudge the base time forward by another fifteen minutes. And do as before. If at any stage he sleeps past the base time, do not wake him to feed. He has nudged his base time forward all on his own! Simply create a new base time straight away – the one he sleeps to, as he has shown he can sleep for that long without needing to be fed: trust him.

Your aim is to nudge the night feed forward until it disappears altogether and your baby is sleeping through to the morning.

Remember that if you ever have problems calming or distracting your baby while he is waiting for his feed, it is fine to pick him up, rock him or cuddle him, and if at any stage you think he is genuinely hungry before his base time and cannot wait, you can feed him and bring the base time earlier for a couple of days before reverting to where you were before. You should never feel uncomfortable following this technique.

So what happens during the rest of the night? In the first few weeks a baby who is fed between 2.30 and 3.30 will probably need a second feed around three hours later. But as with the main feed, try not to feed him before he needs to be fed. Use spaced soothing to get you there if necessary.

It is not a good idea to give your baby a full feed for his second night-time feed or he will not be hungry for his first daytime feed, which follows soon after. Here is a rough guide. If your baby's base time is 2.30 a.m. and he wakes for his second feed between 5 and 5.30 a.m., use spaced soothing to keep him going until 5.30 a.m. (three hours later). Then give him half a feed. You can either dilute a bottle feed with 50 per cent water, give a short feed on the breast, or give a reduced amount of breastmilk from a bottle (or you could dilute it with water). If he waits until 5.30 to 6 a.m. give him a quarter of a feed.

By the time your baby is sleeping happily until after 6 a.m. he is very close to sleeping all the way from his middle-of-the-night feed to 7 a.m. There is little point in a second feed now and your best option is to do spaced soothing until 7 a.m. or to bring the 7 a.m. feed forward a bit for a few days only. You must resist the temptation to get your baby up early or he will start to think that every day starts early and get very grumpy if you don't share his enthusiasm one day. He needs to learn to sleep until 7 a.m.

Once this second feed disappears, you will be left with just the middle-of-the-night feed which you will stretch bit by bit until it too disappears. It gets easier the closer you get. Take heart from this story of a mum who managed this with three babies:

> 'For what seemed like weeks, two of my boys were sleeping until 3 a.m. with us unable to stretch them further. I began to feel desperate as well as exhausted. Then one night I took the bull by the horns, and decided to pace the room with a baby in my arms to make him wait the fifteen minutes extra time to stretch him. It was worth it: we were on a roll. The feed times raced forward. It took only two weeks for the boys to sleep through to 7 a.m. – they were fourteen weeks. Thank God I persevered. They are now eighteen months old and they sleep like . . . babies!'
> **Lidia, mother of triplets**

One day you really will wake up to realize that your baby has slept through to the morning. Hooray!

I am worried I won't be able to do this

Although it takes just a few weeks to get a baby sleeping well, it can seem longer when you take each sleep-interrupted night at a time. In those unforgiving small hours of the morning you can feel as if you are destined for a life of no sleep. Many parents give up on this technique after a few days because results aren't instantaneous. They pick their baby up at every grumble he makes, take him out of the bedroom to distract him, feed him even if he's not hungry, even let him sleep in their bed so that everyone can get some rest.

None of these things makes you a bad parent. But what you cannot achieve by doing this is to teach your baby to sleep well. Sleeping through the night will remain an elusive dream – if only you could get to sleep long enough to have that dream . . .

It may be trite, but it really is a case of 'short-term pain, long-term gain'. Leaving this until a later date will be no easier. If you start this process when your baby is just a couple of weeks old you can be sure of having a full night's sleep in only eight weeks' time. Followed, of course, by many years of the same.

Dropping the dream feed

Once your baby is sleeping from 11 p.m. to 7 a.m. you can start the last phase – the icing on the cake: working towards a full twelve hours of uninterrupted sleep by dropping the dream feed. All being well, you'll find this easier than you think.

The first thing you should do is stop changing your baby's nappy before the dream feed. You no longer want to wake him too much at this time.

When your baby has slept soundly from 11 p.m. to 7 a.m. for a week, bring the dream feed forward by fifteen minutes to 10.45 p.m. If he still sleeps until seven the next morning – and does so for at least three nights – bring the dream feed forward by another fifteen minutes to 10.30 p.m. If he wakes early now, use spaced soothing to get him through to 7 a.m. Once he has managed that for three nights bring the feed forward to 10.15 p.m. Do the same until the dream feed is at 10 p.m. When your baby has slept until seven the next morning for three nights, cut the dream feed altogether.

Don't worry if your baby is not taking a full feed while you are doing this. It could be a good sign that he is ready to let this feed go.

Many parents keep the dream feed going for longer than they need, because they worry that they will disrupt what they have worked hard to achieve, namely an unbroken night's sleep. The disruption rarely happens: if a baby wakes earlier in the morning it should take only a couple of days of spaced soothing to get him back on track and sleeping through until about 7 a.m.

There are other options for dropping the dream feed. You could bring it forward to 10.30 (rather than 10.45) for a week, and then 10 p.m. for another week before dropping it altogether. Or you could ditch all these gradual approaches and simply drop the dream feed one night. You may be pleasantly surprised at the outcome.

Yes, you are there. You have a baby who can sleep through the night. If he can do it once he can do it time and again. Congratulations!

Do I have to start this when my baby is small or can I delay?

These techniques will work with a baby of any age up until about six months, but after that it does become harder. The key, though, is for you to feel ready when you start, and if you are not ready at the beginning it is fine to wait a while until you are. The earlier you start, the earlier your baby will learn to sleep through the night and the sooner everyone can benefit.

And without wishing to alarm you – but in case you are thinking of taking a chance that your baby will learn to sleep through the night of his own accord – studies suggest that a third of all babies still wake at least once a night at the age of six months. Which is not a fun prospect . . .

The next chapter will provide you with some answers to the more detailed questions you might have along the way as you use this method.

The night-time technique

7 p.m.: *Bedtime ritual*
Bath or top 'n' tail
Music
Massage
Dress
Treat every hour now as night-time
Lower lights, avoid talking, avoid eye contact
Feed and wind
Swaddle
Lay baby in cot awake
Music off, lights out
If baby doesn't settle, check for wind or hunger
If he still doesn't settle, use spaced soothing until he falls asleep
Don't rush to your baby at every sound.

11 p.m.: Give your baby his *dream feed*
(this may be a little earlier in the first couple of weeks)
Wake gently, change nappy
Keep lights low, avoid talking, avoid eye contact
Feed and wind
Lay baby in cot awake
Lights out
If baby doesn't settle, check for wind and hunger

If he still doesn't settle, use spaced soothing until he falls asleep

Don't rush to your baby at every sound.

If your baby wakes, use spaced soothing until his base time

Feed, keep lights low, avoid talking, avoid eye contact

No need to change nappy unless it is dirty

Settle

If baby doesn't settle, check for wind and hunger

If he still doesn't settle, use spaced soothing until he falls asleep

When baby has slept to his base time for three days out of five nudge the base time on by fifteen minutes to stretch his sleep until he sleeps through the night. If at any stage he sleeps past the base time do not wake him. Use his new waking time as the new base time.

Second reduced feed if needed (around three hours after base time)

Keep lights low, avoid talking, avoid eye contact

No need to change nappy unless it is dirty

Settle

If baby doesn't settle, use spaced soothing until he falls asleep

Wake baby at around 7 a.m. and give him his first full feed of the day

If he wakes before this time use spaced soothing until he falls asleep – or to keep him calm and distracted until the day begins and he can get up

When baby sleeps from the dream feed to 7 a.m., prepare to drop the dream feed.

For feeding quantities check the chart on p. 86.

10.

Problem-solving at Night

'Now that you are working on getting your baby to sleep through the night, a helping hand may not come amiss – just in case things don't work out exactly as you had expected. After all, even the best-laid plans can encounter the occasional hitch and I too find that babies sometimes do things I'm not expecting.

'So if you come up against a problem don't think you're doing things wrong, are a bad parent or have any reason to give up on your attempts to help your baby to sleep. It's just that it can take time. All you need is a little patience and perhaps a bit of guidance. Which is what this chapter will provide.'

Jo

The first six weeks

What if . . .

My two-week-old baby won't take more than an ounce of milk at 11 p.m. however hard I try.

Newborns are often very sleepy at this time which is why it's important to change their nappy before this feed as this helps to wake them up. You could also try laying your baby on the bed unswaddled for a few minutes to make him more alert.

Remember, you don't need to wind your baby during this feed

as he may fall asleep while the breast or bottle is not in his mouth and you'll have trouble getting it back in. Wait until the end of the feed.

My three-week-old baby is screaming an hour after I put him to bed at 7 p.m. even though he's been settling well for the last couple of weeks.
The culprits at this time of night are usually wind or hunger. If you are breastfeeding and had a suspicion that your milk supply was a little low when you fed him at 7 p.m. (as many mums find), offer him longer on the breast, or the second breast, or give him a top-up feed of expressed milk or formula. If you think your baby may have wind, you can start using an over-the-counter remedy which may be effective. You will need to give it before every feed for several days.

If you have checked for wind and hunger and your baby is still unsettled, check for a dirty nappy. Your baby may simply be overtired, which can make it harder for him to fall asleep.

If you have been doing spaced soothing for an hour and he's still screaming there may be another reason, such as colic or constipation (see chapter 11). If this screaming continues for more than a couple of nights and you can't pinpoint what is troubling your baby, you might want to see your doctor.

Very young babies, under about four weeks old, cannot calm themselves without help when they are upset, so it's best to pick them up and cuddle them. Use a dummy if you find this soothes your baby. Remember always to put him in his cot before he falls asleep.

My three-week-old baby wakes at 9.30 p.m. and won't wait until 11 p.m. to be fed.
Young babies, and especially low-birthweight babies, can only go for three hours at the most between feeds. Give him a small feed and then his full feed at 11 p.m. If he's over 7 lb you can start to

use spaced soothing to stretch this small feed by ten to fifteen minutes every few days until it reaches the 11 p.m. dream feed. If not, wait until he is.

If your baby is a good healthy weight and took a full feed at 7 p.m., it's unlikely that he's waking through hunger. If you've noticed that this is a pattern and you have been responding by giving him milk, it could be that he's simply got used to waking for food at 9.30: babies quickly develop internal 'alarm clocks'.

To get him back on track, do spaced soothing for up to about fifteen minutes. If he still hasn't settled, try a very small feed. Then settle him, but wake him again at 11 p.m. for his full feed. If the same happens the following night wait a little longer before giving him a small feed, maybe a total of twenty minutes or so, and a little longer the night after. After about seven days he should be back on track and sleeping until 11 p.m.

My three-week-old baby hates having a massage and I'm wondering if I have to do this to make the bedtime ritual work.
Of course you don't. At three weeks he is probably a little young to enjoy a massage.

Massage isn't everyone's cup of tea, and is certainly no fun if you or your baby are tense or unhappy, but it's worth persisting with because massage time often becomes one of the best bits of your and your baby's day, though not until you are both ready for it. Just try again in a couple of weeks and see if your baby starts to enjoy it.

Your baby might not like being naked when you are massaging, so make sure he is covered everywhere you are not actually massaging to keep him warm.

My four-week-old baby sleeps happily in his rocker chair during the day but seems to hate his cot.
Try putting your baby in his cot (awake) during the day with his

mobile playing while you potter around the room. You could swaddle him at night (until he is about six weeks old) to make him feel secure. If he has been sleeping in a moses basket then put this inside the cot for a week so he gets used to the new surroundings.

My four-week-old baby has been constipated and has been screaming every time I lay him down. He's had some cooled boiled water, has done a poo and is much happier but I am wondering what to do if this happens again. Should I keep following your guidelines or comfort him and cuddle him to sleep?
Whenever a baby is unwell or in pain you should always do what you feel is best for your baby. If that means you want to comfort him and cuddle him until he's calm that's absolutely fine. Try using a dummy when he goes to bed as this may soothe him but take it out before he is in a deep sleep (see p. 201 on constipation).

Try to stick as closely as you can to his normal feed and sleep times and don't worry – you won't throw out your plans to get your baby to sleep well provided the cuddling doesn't become a habit when it isn't needed.

I am breastfeeding my four-week-old baby and she takes most of her feed in ten minutes, so how can I give her a reduced feed for her second night-time feed in the night?
A reduced feed is helpful when your baby needs to be fed between about five or 6 a.m. but you don't want to spoil the first feed of the morning. You could try giving her just a couple of ounces of expressed milk, or even dilute it with a little cooled boiled water.

My four-week-old baby has been waking at 3 a.m. every night for two weeks and I am using this as his base time. He won't sleep past it though, so how can I set a new base time?
Try to make him wait fifteen minutes for his feed. Use spaced soothing to help you do this. You may find that he falls asleep before the

fifteen minutes are up and wakes later, which becomes your new base time. If he doesn't, feed him at 3.15 and do the same the following night. Within a few days (seven at the most) he will be able to go until 3.15, which is your new base time, and in a few days you can start to nudge the time on by another quarter of an hour.

'Sandra's baby was four weeks old and following my night-time techniques to get her feeds stretched and sleeping through. She was doing so well. Amy was sleeping through until 3.45 a.m. and was obviously on the way to sleeping through the night at an early age.

'But then she started to wake at 2 a.m. and demanded to be fed. Sandra looked at her log and realized that because Amy was sleepy she had been having only half a feed at 4 p.m. and was obviously missing out and getting hungry. Sandra made her take a full feed at that time, increased all her feeds by five minutes on the breast and offered Amy a top-up of expressed breastmilk at the 7 p.m. feed. Within three days she was sleeping until 4 a.m.'

Jo

Six weeks to four months

What if . . .

My six-week-old baby doesn't like sleeping on his back.
Some babies seem to be more comfortable sleeping on their tummies, but as this can be a factor implicated in cot death it's not recommended. Your baby may settle for lying on his side. Roll up a small blanket and put it behind your baby's back (not behind his head) to prop him and make sure his lower arm is extended so he can't turn on to his front.

'Tania's eleven-week-old twins wouldn't sleep on their backs and needed to be rocked or given a dummy to settle. At eleven weeks they were still waking frequently during the night. They no longer needed feeding but did need a dummy and Tania was worried that they were becoming dependent on it. They were waking at 6 a.m. for a feed but then refusing to go back to sleep.

'The first thing I suggested to Tania was to stop using dummies during the day as the first step towards weaning the twins off them. I also showed her how to put the boys to sleep on their sides. We then put them to sleep on their backs at the afternoon naps and after the dream feed as they were always very tired at those times. We used spaced soothing if they started to cry, and if they got very upset we would switch them to their side. But after only three days they got used to the idea of sleeping on their backs and never again complained.

'The early-morning waking was down to sunlight streaming through the windows so we got blackout blinds fitted.

'When the boys woke during the night we slowly replaced the dummies with simple soothing – stroking their noses and calming them with ssshhhhhh sounds. After nine days they were waking only briefly at night and settling themselves back to sleep. They woke again at 6.30 but would fall asleep a few minutes later without a feed.

'Tania noticed how much more cheerful the boys were once they slept well. Her husband noticed how much more cheerful Tania was too!'

Jo

My six-week-old baby wakes at 2.30 a.m. every night. (I have been feeding him and he has gone straight back to sleep.)

If your baby was born at a good weight (above 7 lb) he should be able to sleep longer than three and a half hours at night by the age of six weeks. Many parents assume that because their baby falls asleep after a feed he must have been hungry, so they carry on feeding at the same time every night. What happens though is that their baby starts to rely on a feed to sleep.

Check the feed chart to see if your baby is getting enough milk during the day and don't forget to give him his dream feed at 11 p.m. Parents are sometimes tempted to miss this out because they and their baby are sleepy at this time, but it's very important to stick with it.

Next time your baby wakes, leave him for a few minutes before doing spaced soothing to help him settle back to sleep. If after about fifteen minutes he won't settle, you could give him a small feed (a breastfeed or a diluted formula feed), then put him back in his cot. Do this for five nights but give him a tiny bit less milk each night. After the fifth night just do spaced soothing and with luck he will soon start to sleep longer.

I'm too tired to do spaced soothing so I sometimes leave my six-week-old baby to cry without going to him and he usually goes back to sleep.

Leaving your baby to cry until he settles himself to sleep will do him no harm, so please don't worry. But don't leave your baby crying for more than fifteen minutes. Some parents don't feel strong enough to do this, but many who use the spaced soothing technique for a few weeks find they develop the confidence to leave their baby a little longer before going to him, knowing that it can help him to fall asleep on his own.

My seven-week-old baby was sleeping through to his base time at 4.15 but has started to wake again at 2.15 and I am wondering what I have done wrong.

You have done nothing wrong. Sometimes babies will revert to waking a little earlier but this will probably last only a few days. Learning to sleep through the night takes a while and there are steps backward as well as steps forward along the way.

Check the chart to see if he is getting enough milk during the day. Try not to feed him when he wakes at 2.15 but do spaced soothing for as long as you can and give him a dummy if it helps.

My eight-week-old baby is sleeping six hours during the day – could this be why he is waking in the middle of the night?

Yes, it could well be affecting his night-time sleep. Check the sleep chart to see roughly how much sleep your baby needs during the day and try to bring it down a little at each of the naps. But don't be tempted to let your baby get overtired in the hope that he will sleep better. Overtired babies find it hard to sleep.

I started following your night-time techniques when my baby was eight weeks old but after three days of things going well I did spaced soothing for two hours in the middle of the night and I am wondering if this is normal.

This can happen but won't last long. The third and fourth days of doing things a new way are often the toughest. This is when some people give up, not realizing perhaps that it takes time for a baby to break existing habits and adjust to something different. If you give up now your baby will get confused; when you try again later he may suspect you won't see it through. Try to stick at it, for your baby's sake. It usually takes a baby about seven days to learn a new way of doing things, so you are not far away.

My eight-week-old baby slept from 11 p.m. to 6.30 three nights ago and I was over the moon. I thought we had got there. But since then she has reverted to waking at 5 a.m. What have I done wrong?

You have done nothing wrong. It is not uncommon for a baby to do this. The fact that your baby slept for so long one night is a good sign that she is on the way to doing so every night. Eight weeks is still a little early for a baby to sleep an eight-hour stretch every night but it will happen soon. Don't give up – you are so close.

My ten-week-old baby has colic and I find it hard to do anything after 5.30 that follows your routine.

Colic is very distressing for both parents and their babies. It usually starts late in the afternoon and persists until some time around midnight. (There are some ideas on p. 197 on what you can do to help a colicky baby.)

It is true that it is harder to get a baby with colic into a routine and sleeping through the night but colic disappears at around fourteen weeks. Until then it's a good idea to follow the routine as far as you can, and to follow the bedtime ritual as closely as possible. That way, when the colic disappears your baby will already know and understand the routine. Sometimes babies with colic have problems sleeping after the colic has gone for the simple reason that their parents have become accustomed to rushing to them at every cry: these babies have never learned to fall asleep on their own. The parents, who by then are exhausted, assume all is lost by the time the colic has disappeared and don't try to get a bedtime routine going. But it's never too late to start.

My ten-week-old baby won't take more than an ounce at 11 p.m. however hard I try.

As babies get older they reach a point where the amount they drink at 11 p.m. has little effect on how long they sleep. This is usually when they are close to sleeping through from 11 p.m. to

7 a.m. (which can be any time after about ten weeks) and is a sign that they will soon not need this feed any more. When your baby sleeps from 7 p.m. to 11 p.m. and then 11 p.m. to 7 a.m. for a week you can drop the 11 p.m. dream feed.

My ten-week-old baby is waking at 4.30 in the morning and won't fall back to sleep until about 6 a.m.
Check that your baby's room is dark and check for any noises that may be intruding regularly at this time. Look at the sleep chart to see whether your baby is sleeping too much during the day.

Try spaced soothing when he wakes and when he is calm, leave him. He may simply be craving your attention: if you keep offering it he may start to expect it every night; if you don't, he'll soon get bored and fall asleep. If he gets upset and spaced soothing doesn't calm him, pick him up and cuddle him and when he quietens put him down awake. You should find that after a few days of doing this he will sleep past 4.30.

My baby was sleeping from 11 p.m. until 7 a.m. for a few days but now wakes at 5.30 and seems to think the day has started.
Don't be tempted to let your baby decide that this is when all his days are going to start. Otherwise you will all be exhausted very soon.

Check the sleep chart to see whether your baby is sleeping too much in the day.

Babies have a phase of light sleep in the early hours and if there is noise or light there's a chance they may wake up. That's why blackout blinds are so helpful, especially in summer. See if you can identify a particular noise that may be waking him (is it dad getting up to go to work?). You can either try spaced soothing to encourage your baby back to sleep, or if he is not unhappy at being awake, and if you feel comfortable doing so, you could leave him. He may not fall asleep straight away, but after a few days of doing this he will probably settle himself back to sleep quite quickly or start sleeping through.

I took my eight-week-old baby into my bed at 6 a.m. this morning because he wouldn't settle and now I am worried I have done the wrong thing.

No, you haven't done the wrong thing. If you want to give your baby some reassurance and comfort by taking him into your bed now and then, why shouldn't you? You're his mum! And it's comforting for you too. If you don't want this to become a habit, then try to limit how often you do it, so your baby doesn't get hooked on the idea.

My baby is now three months old and is sleeping through the night but I am worried he will not be getting as much milk as he needs.

Don't worry. Your baby will make up for it during his daytime feeds.

My baby is fourteen weeks old and sleeping from 11 p.m. to 7 a.m. However, I have just tried to drop his dream feed and he has started waking at 2.30 again – I am in despair.

Don't despair. This does not happen very often but when it does it is usually with babies who are still drinking large amounts at the dream feed. The majority of babies of this age want only a small feed at 11 p.m. and this is a good sign that they are ready to give up their dream feed.

Reintroduce the dream feed and over the course of a week reduce the amount that you give your baby. Once he is taking no more than a small feed try dropping it again.

My baby is four months old, doesn't sleep through the night and I've only just bought this book. Will it help me?

Yes it will, although it can be a little harder to get your baby used to a night-time routine now. Your baby is already capable of sleeping through the night at this age but it may take at least a week for him to learn to do so and you will need to be very determined to stick at it. Babies of this age have acquired habits and patterns that need to be changed; that will take time. But if you are consistent and see the process through, it will work.

'Marco was five months old and waking almost every hour through the night. His mother, Susan, would then feed him, rock him to sleep or take him into her bed, which she wasn't comfortable about. She was exhausted.

'I showed her the night-time settling techniques and within a week Marco was sleeping through the night. Susan was over the moon, not just because she was able to sleep herself but also because of the changes she noticed in Marco. She realized that she had been rushing to him too soon, whenever he grumbled or cried, and that had prevented him from learning to fall asleep on his own.

'This is the sleep log of Marco's progress.'
Jo

Marco's sleep log

Night 1
Marco woke eight times.
    Went to him to do spaced soothing a total of sixteen times.

Night 2
Marco woke six times.
    Went to him and did spaced soothing four times.

Night 3
Marco woke once.

Didn't go in to him as he settled back to sleep on his own.

Night 4
Marco woke five times.
  Went to him and did spaced soothing five times.

Night 5
Marco woke four times.
  Went to him and did spaced soothing four times.

Night 6
Marco woke twice.
  Didn't need to go to him as he settled back to sleep on his own.

Night 7
Marco woke once.
  Didn't have to go to him because he settled back to sleep on his own.

'I had seriously been wondering if there was something wrong with Marco. I had been to specialist paediatricians, osteopaths, etc. but Jo's techniques and subsequent results proved that he simply wasn't getting enough proper rest. I distinctly remember putting him down to bed for the night after Jo had gone and his kicking three times (happily) and smiling. He pretty much still does that when he goes to bed, a year on. The best thing for me was seeing a whingey, miserable baby become not only tolerable but enjoyable to have around.'
Susan

My baby is five months old and has started to roll on to his tummy at night but then can't roll back.

He will soon be able to roll himself back. Until he does, turn him over calmly and quietly and then leave him to settle. Some babies roll over deliberately if they think it will get them some attention; others simply do so because they like it.

My baby is six months old and has slept really well from around three months of age. But just recently he has started to wake at 4 a.m.

Some babies who start to sleep well from an early age subsequently go through a phase of night waking at around six to twelve months. It is nearly always a passing phase, so don't despair. Teething is occasionally the cause of the waking, as is hunger. Review how much you are feeding during the day. Another reason could be that at this age babies may go through intense dreaming phases from which they wake abruptly. It could also be that, if your baby is still sharing your room, he wants attention. Now may be the time to consider moving him to his own room.

General

What if . . .

I would rather work on getting my baby to sleep through the night when he is a little older as I feel this is all a bit too soon.

It is really never too early for a baby to sleep well and to benefit from doing so. If you want to leave it until later you will all get overtired. Sleep deprivation can be very tough to cope with.

You will also run the risk that in the meantime your baby may develop bad sleep habits which will stay with him for some time. Babies and young children don't, as a rule, simply grow out of sleep problems. They can become toddlers who don't sleep, even young children who don't sleep.

As a baby gets older it can be much harder to teach him to sleep well. Take heed of this story:

> '*Molly was still sleeping in our bed when she was two and a half because we had no idea how to get her to sleep on her own. By then we knew we had to do something, so we started controlled crying with her but it was absolutely hideous, just awful. We did it for a week, but when we went on holiday we couldn't bear it, so we gave up.*
>
> '*We didn't have the energy to try again until she was four and this time it was impossible. She would cry out for us and sob. At that age children don't give in easily. So we gave in and she came back into our bed. We never had any evenings to ourselves — she would be up and about after a couple of hours wanting us to come to bed. She had developed a fear of being on her own. She ended up sleeping in our bed until she was six.*
>
> '*I would urge any parent not to let this happen. We nearly made the same mistake with our second child and I do not know how I would have coped. To this day I thank my lucky stars that we met Jo and she helped us to get him sleeping through when he was still a baby.*'
> **Julie**

This is what you can hope for instead:

> '*Thanks to Jo our first baby, Lidia, slept through the night in her own bed from seven to seven at the age of eleven weeks. She's now three and she still sleeps wonderfully. I'm sure this is because she learned to sleep well from such an early age. When her younger sister, Amaya, arrived Jo got her to sleep through the night by eight weeks and she still does so at the age of eighteen months. Now my friends*

*can't believe I have two small children who sleep so well.
We hardly ever have a broken night, we get our evenings to
ourselves and we get our sleep – which we need with two
toddlers.'*
Annabel

I can't settle my baby after the middle-of-the-night feed.
This can happen with babies of any age. Maybe there's a little bit
of trapped wind? Lift your baby up (this often brings out stubborn
wind), and then put him back in his cot and try to let him settle
himself. You could place him on his side, with his lower arm
extended to stop him rolling over on to his tummy. This should
soothe him and help him to drift off.

If he still grumbles he may just be trying to settle himself. The
best thing you can do is to reassure him that you are there with
spaced soothing, but to leave him to fall asleep alone. Remember,
babies make a lot of noises when they wind down.

*I am worried that if my baby sleeps through the night my breastmilk
will start to dry up.*
Please don't worry. Your body will adapt to producing all the
milk your baby needs at whatever time of night or day it's needed;
it will simply adjust to your baby's new feeding pattern. The extra
sleep you will get will help to keep your milk supply up.

*I worry that my baby will become too dependent on his dummy
because I've been using it to soothe him.*
Parents often worry about using dummies, but they are a great
help for calming a baby during the day and helping him to settle
himself to sleep at night, during the early months. (See p. 38 for
a discussion on dummies.)

If you don't want your baby's dummy to become a permanent
fixture then you might plan to wean him off it at around the

four-month mark. Start by taking it away during the day and remove it at night only once your baby is sleeping through. This might be a bit of a challenge for the first couple of nights and your baby may need extra soothing. But it shouldn't last long: many parents are pleasantly surprised at how quickly their baby settles himself to sleep without a dummy once it has been removed.

You could give your baby a muslin with a knot tied in the middle (so it can't drape across your baby's face). Your baby may grab it or even suck on it, taking his mind off the vanishing dummy.

I have a feeling that my baby is crying because he's learned that spaced soothing means I will always go in after only five minutes.
Maybe we underestimate how clever babies are. It's quite possible that your baby has worked out how to get your attention and if this worries you, you could vary the times before you go to him, say seven minutes followed by five minutes and then perhaps ten. He will still feel reassured to know that you are there if he needs you.

I have a feeling that my baby gets agitated when I do spaced soothing because he can smell my breastmilk.
Mums do sometimes find this happens. One way around the problems is to get dad to do the spaced soothing, and if necessary the middle-of-the-night feeds with a bottle of expressed milk or formula.

I left my baby to cry for longer than the recommended five minutes last night because I was so tired and he fell back asleep. Have I done any harm?
Parents sometimes remark that when they leave their baby for a little longer than five minutes he falls asleep without their needing

to soothe him. Some parents will even do so time and again; it is highly unlikely that this could cause a baby any trauma. If it feels right for you, that is fine.

11.

Minor Ailments and Upsets

'All parents are paranoid about their babies' health – and who can blame us when our babies seem so frail and vulnerable? I worried myself silly at the sight of the tiniest spot or at the slightest snuffle when mine were small.

'As time went on I learned that most babies are more resilient than we sometimes imagine. But I've also learned never to feel embarrassed or awkward about calling a doctor or going to Accident and Emergency if I am worried. When one of my boys swallowed a plum stone I phoned my GP and had him call the consultant at the local hospital for advice. (The advice was to wait until the stone appeared at the other end . . .) It didn't matter how stupid I felt.

'But for those grumbles that don't automatically need a doctor's input, this guide to the most common, and relatively minor, baby ailments will help. And there are some ideas too on the things that we mums and our bodies go through after childbirth.'
Barbara

'Please remember these tips are not a substitute for medical advice and don't apply to serious illnesses. When your baby is still under three months you should *always* seek medical advice if he has a fever, vomiting or diarrhoea. And go with your instincts: if you think there is

something wrong with your baby, act on it. Don't feel you won't be heard.'
Jo

Baby ailments

Baby's bits

Sometimes, a few days after birth, both boys and girls develop slightly swollen breasts. This is the effect of the surge in mum's hormones at birth: they pass through to the baby. Girls may also have a slightly blood-tinged vaginal discharge.

Belly button stump (the umbilical cord)

The stump remaining from the umbilical cord usually dries up and breaks away around ten days after birth, leaving a small wound which soon heals. Until it does, keep the stump clean and dry. Use saline solution to clean it and pat it dry with a towel or a tissue. You could use medicated talc if it seeps, and if it gets red or pussy, consult your midwife or health visitor. Keep the top of your baby's nappy folded if there's any chance of it rubbing.

Blood in nappy

Brown, pink or red stains in a newborn's nappy are caused by urates in the urine and are completely normal. Talk to your midwife if you are concerned.

A baby of any age can contract a urinary tract infection which may cause blood in the urine and can be accompanied by a fever. This is serious and requires immediate treatment, usually in hospital.

Bottle blisters

Babies sometimes get a blister on their top lip from sucking a bottle or breastfeeding; it usually drops off but may then re-form. It's nothing to worry about.

Colds

Babies often get the snuffles, even if they're breastfed.

Try steam: take your baby into a steamy bathroom for about fifteen minutes or invest in a warm-air humidifier to release water vapour throughout the day and night.

You could stroke the inside of your baby's nostril gently with a tiny bit of cotton wool to encourage him to sneeze and clear the mucus. If this doesn't work, try putting saline drops in your baby's nose first to help thin out the mucus, wait a couple of minutes and then aspirate with a nasal aspirator (sold in pharmacies). You can buy saline drops in a small bottle or make your own (half a teaspoon of salt to 8 oz water – no stronger). Keep the solution in a sterile bottle and throw it away after a week. Use a cotton wool ball soaked in the mixture to drop one to two drops into each nostril, or use a sterile eye-dropper. Do this before your baby feeds or it may make him vomit.

Don't use anything containing menthol on your baby before he is three months as it can irritate the delicate nose lining. You can, though, place some Vicks Baby Balsam in a bowl of boiling water and put it in his room. After three months you can use decongestant oils or creams.

To help him breathe more easily, raise your baby's head very slightly by placing a small pillow under one end of the mattress. But if there is any sign that your baby is having difficulty breathing you must contact a doctor.

Colic

Colic is very distressing – not just for your baby, but for you too. It usually starts when babies are around two to three weeks old and invariably disappears at about three months, which is something to keep at the front of your mind in your lowest moments. It's unclear exactly what causes colic but it's generally thought to be the result of an immature digestive system.

Babies with colic usually start to cry in the late afternoon. The crying is distinctive – a high-pitched squeal – and a baby may also draw his legs up and become very red in the face. The cries can subside, lulling you into believing the pain has gone away, only for the crying to start again. Some babies cry into the night, which is very tough on everyone.

Frequent breastfeeds are sometimes recommended but may make the pain worse as frequent gulping can build up wind, and too much foremilk may contribute to colic. You could try Infacol to bring out the wind circulating in your baby's tummy, or Colief, which is specifically designed for babies with colic and breaks down the lactose in milk, making it more digestible. Your baby may find relief from a dummy: sucking calms babies.

If you are breastfeeding, you could drink chamomile or fennel tea and you could even try giving a few drops to your baby too.

Your baby may get relief if you hold him in one of the following two positions:

The lazy rabbit: Sit down and lay your baby across your legs on his tummy. Keep his legs slightly lower than his head to stop any milk coming up.

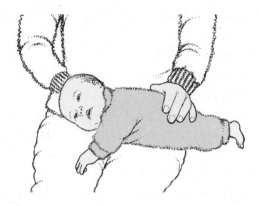

Tiger in a tree: Hold your baby along your forearm, facing down, with his head resting near your elbow and your hand on his tummy. Use your other arm to support your baby in this position and keep him close to your body. The pressure and warmth from your hand around his tummy should soothe him.

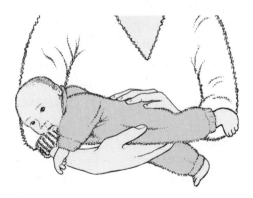

Colic can make it hard to establish a bedtime routine, but it is still worth trying to follow one. At around 5.30 p.m., when colic usually starts, you could give your baby a small top-up feed or a couple of ounces of cooled boiled water. This should settle his tummy. A bath in the evening will help to soothe and distract him. Try a massage after the bath, massaging his tummy in a clockwise direction. Feed him in his bedroom as usual, swaddle him if you can and give him a dummy. You may find that putting your baby down on his side will help ease his pain. If he is not swaddled, extend his lower arm so he doesn't roll over on to his tummy. If he is, support him with a rolled-up blanket behind his back.

Put your baby to bed as you usually would. You will probably have to keep returning to him to comfort him but try not to take him out of the darkened bedroom when you do so, as it will confuse him about night and day. Despite his discomfort, he is still able to learn the difference between daytime and night-time.

Many parents with colicky babies find cranial osteopathy is a godsend. The theory of this treatment is that a baby's skull plates – which are soft and not yet fused – sometimes become slightly misaligned at birth (or in the womb) through the pressure exerted on them. This can cause stresses on the whole body including the central nervous system and can contribute to colic (as well as a number of other problems such as sleep disturbances, feeding difficulties, constant crying, sickness and wind).

The treatment involves the very gentlest of pressure on the baby's head and neck to correct the misalignments. If you are sceptical about this you might like to know that two recent small studies carried out in the UK have shown that cranial osteopathic treatment is effective in reducing the amount of crying in colicky babies as well as improving their sleeping (see Notes, p. 289).

'Colic may be distressing for a baby but it's also all extremely distressing for parents, and even more so in the case of twins, as there's never the opportunity for mum and dad to take turns standing in the garden for half an hour with their hands over their ears, weeping with exhaustion.

'This was the situation we found ourselves in with our twin girls, Florence and Isabella. It started around six in the evening, often went on for five or six hours and was a daily torture for all four of us. They would suffer the most excruciating writhing agonies, arching their backs, bending double and screaming the house down.

'We tried every remedy we came across: various gripe waters, syrups, milk additives . . . but nothing worked. Then we read an article about cranial osteopathy.

'Our osteopath asked us about the girls and in particular their positions and circumstances of birth. Florence had been the lower of the two, and breech, and Isabella had been pushing on her head for the last few weeks of the pregnancy. (The girls were born by caesarean, five weeks early.) The osteopath suggested that Florence's spinal vertebrae at the top of her neck may have been compressed during the third trimester, and that the resulting misalignment of the vertebrae was a very common cause of discomfort or pain (and colic) in young children. Even single babies could have the same problem as a result of the way their heads lay bent in the womb, and it could take months or years for the problem to sort itself out. In fact, she suggested that some adults who suffered from back or neck pain in later life could trace the causes of their problems right back to the way their necks were bent before birth.

'The treatment was to lay the baby on the bed and gently apply fingertips to the base of the skull, in order to release some of the pressure on the vertebrae and assist the alignment of the spine. Even watching carefully, it was impossible to observe any obvious pressure or movement on the part of the osteopath. I felt as though we were watching an Antiques Roadshow expert handling a *priceless artefact, so slow and gentle were the movements. Any fears that there might be inappropriate force applied to such a tiny and fragile neck were quickly allayed.*

'During the sessions, each baby would visibly relax. For some time afterwards it was clear that there was a deeply soothing effect, and within two to three weeks the awful symptoms of colic subsided. Whether this was a coincidence of timing or cause and effect, we could not be sure. What was certain, though, was that the treatment seemed to soothe the babies for a while. For us, the experience of having someone give such tender attention to the children and to sit in such a quiet and peaceful place was valuable in itself.'

Dan

It's also worth trying cranial osteopathy if your baby is distressed, irritable or just unsettled for no clear or obvious reason. More and more parents are turning to this treatment for their babies and you should be able to find a practitioner in your area.

Constipation

Many babies grunt, groan and generally strain when having a poo so the only way to tell if your baby is constipated is by his stools. If there are fewer than one a day and/or it is hard and pellet-like, it's likely your baby is constipated.

Constipation is generally more likely in babies who are bottle-fed. (It's not uncommon for babies to become constipated later when they move on to solid foods.)

If there's no sign of a poo after twenty-four hours give your baby an ounce of cooled boiled water, fifteen to thirty minutes before a feed, in the morning. If this doesn't have the desired effect, give him some more the following morning and again before the next two feeds. If after two days of doing this there's still no movement, you can add a teaspoon of prune or fresh orange juice (strained and with no pulp) to the water. This usually works within hours.

It's best to give the water in the morning so it can take effect during the day and be dealt with. You may also find that bicycling your baby's legs will give him some relief.

Cradle cap

This can look much worse than it is. At best a baby's scalp seems to have bad dandruff, at worst it becomes covered with a greasy, flaky yellow crust. Sometimes it spreads to the eyebrows and behind the ears. It's unsightly but is quite common and won't cause any irritation. Cradle cap seems to be the result of a build-up of oils on the skin and usually affects babies between about two and six months of age.

You can try to prevent an outbreak by wiping your baby's scalp in a circular motion with cotton wool and warm water after you shampoo his hair. This will stimulate the blood supply to the scalp and help to avoid a build-up of dead skin. If this doesn't prevent cradle cap, dab baby oil or olive oil on to your baby's scalp and leave it overnight. Shampoo the next morning and the dry skin should lift off. If the problem persists, try the same thing again a couple of days later. If it spreads to the face or neck, or if the skin becomes inflamed, consult your doctor.

Try not to shampoo your baby's hair too often, whether he has cradle cap or not. Three times a week is plenty.

Dehydration

Dehydration is serious and needs urgent medical attention. It can occur through severe vomiting and/or diarrhoea. Some of the signs of dehydration are: dark yellow urine or a succession of dry nappies, dry lips and mouth, a sunken fontanelle (this is the soft spot on the top of your baby's head). A baby will also be weak and unresponsive. Try giving your baby some milk or cooled boiled water while waiting for medical help.

Diarrhoea

You will know your baby has diarrhoea if his stools are very watery (as opposed to loose or a tiny bit runny). If your baby is being breastfed it could be that something you are eating is upsetting your baby's tummy. This can be anything that might cause you wind and could include cauliflower, cabbage, curries, or baked beans. Be sure to keep up your baby's fluid intake, either with milk or, if you think your baby is very thirsty, a small amount of cooled boiled water. If the diarrhoea lasts more than twenty-four hours contact a doctor. If it is accompanied by vomiting it may be gastroenteritis and your baby can get ill very quickly, so call the doctor immediately.

Dry skin

All babies have a tendency towards dry skin, especially around the wrists and ankles. A cheap and effective remedy is aqueous cream (available over the counter at pharmacies), and you can use it on your baby's face if you need to. The cream is also great for massaging your baby but don't use it if your baby has eczema (it may cause stinging). Or you could use grapeseed oil. Very dry skin, on the other hand (and indeed eczema), might need a stronger emollient such as Dipro base cream or Oilatum cream or bath oil (but be careful with the oil as it can make both your baby and your bath very slippery).

For babies under three months it is not necessary to add any baby products to the water. If you feel you want to put something in the bath check that it has no perfume.

If the dry skin doesn't seem to bother your baby you could leave it; it will probably pass.

Eczema

It is common in babies, but can be upsetting for their parents as it can look quite nasty. Eczema usually starts on the face, behind the ears and knees, or in the folds of the neck or elbows.

Your doctor may prescribe a hydrocortisone cream (to use sparingly). Keeping the skin moisturized is very important. If you have been using aqueous cream as a moisturizer, switch to something else such as Dipro base, or even a petroleum jelly, which is messy to apply but very effective. Stop using soap or bubble bath; add Oilatum oil to the bath water instead. Keep your baby's fingernails short so he can't scratch his skin.

Sometimes eczema is a sign that your baby has an intolerance of certain foods, cow's milk being a common one. (In severe cases a dairy intolerance can make a baby bring up cottage cheese-like milk after most feeds and give rise to crusty yellow spots on his face.) As cow's milk is an ingredient in baby formula you could switch to a non-dairy product like goat's milk (or soya) if you are bottle-feeding, but talk to your doctor first. Some mothers have found that reducing their dairy intake, or replacing cow's with goat's milk or soya, helps if they are breastfeeding.

You could also try switching to a non-biological washing powder (if you're not already using one) and stop using fabric conditioner.

Many babies simply grow out of eczema in time.

Gagging

Newborn babies sometimes gag and bring up mucus. This can be alarming but it's just their way of clearing the airways and doesn't last for more than a few days after birth. If it distresses your baby, try placing him on his side when you put him to sleep so any mucus dribbles out of his mouth and doesn't cause him to gag.

Hiccups

Hiccups sound and look dramatic, but are very common in young babies and rarely cause them any distress. They usually start some time after feeding and will go away if you simply wait. If you feel you need to do something, give your baby an ounce of cooled boiled water, or try holding him over your shoulder and patting his back. You don't need to wait for hiccups to stop before putting a baby down to sleep.

Jaundice

More than half of all newborn babies and 80 per cent of pre-term babies develop jaundice two or three days after birth. It can be alarming to see your baby's skin and eyes turn yellow but it causes your baby no discomfort and will disappear after a couple of weeks. Your baby may be given phototherapy treatment under ultra-violet lights (with eye shields to protect his eyes) and you could place him next to a window during the day so he is exposed to daylight.

This will be monitored by your midwife.

Meningitis

Parents understandably worry that spots or a rash may be a sign of meningitis. The Meningitis Research Foundation has a 24-hour helpline (080 8800 3344) as does the Meningitis Trust (0845 6000 800) and can give you advice. If you have any reason to suspect meningitis take your baby straight to your doctor or local hospital.

Nappy rash

You're unlikely to miss nappy rash. Your baby's skin will become red and pimply and may even be inflamed.

The main cause of nappy rash is wetness, and as newborn babies in particular urinate and poo frequently their nappies need regular changing to keep the skin clean and dry. Even if you are meticulous, though, you can't guarantee to keep nappy rash at bay if your baby develops diarrhoea or has very sensitive skin.

In the first two weeks of your baby's life it's best to use cotton wool and warm water on your baby's bottom, rather than baby wipes. Always wipe well in the creases. Dry the skin afterwards with cotton wool or muslin. Change your baby's nappy before each feed and whenever it is dirty. Airing the skin (including nappy-off time once your baby is about four weeks old – see p. 93) even if it's only for five minutes in between changes, is a great preventative.

If a rash starts, air the skin and before putting on a new nappy use some soothing cream or an antiseptic barrier cream.

Reflux

If your baby is sick after every feed, is irritable, cries or screams, arches his back during feeding, wakes frequently at night and is failing to gain weight, he may have gastro-oesophageal reflux. This happens when some of the contents of the stomach move back into the oesophagus. The acid which is brought up is very uncomfortable; if you had heartburn during pregnancy you will know what it is like.

Try propping your baby up for about twenty to thirty minutes after a feed so he can digest his milk more easily. You could even try to feed him in this position. If he refuses to drink, it may be that he is associating drinking with discomfort, so keep persisting and try to get him to take some milk.

Your doctor may suggest an antacid such as Gaviscon which can be given to newborns. Mix it in your baby's milk (use expressed milk and a bottle if you are breastfeeding). Reflux usually goes away once a baby is on solids or is able to sit up on his own.

Sickness

Many babies are sick after a feed, known as possetting, which can be alarming because it seems more than it actually is. If you pour an ounce of milk over a work surface you'll get an idea of how much or how little your baby is actually bringing up. If you think it's too much for comfort, try giving him some cooled boiled water to settle his tummy and wait until his next feed to give him more milk. The water helps his tummy to settle and will prevent dehydration.

If your baby is bringing up far more (vomiting) he will be losing fluids so you need to be sure he doesn't get dehydrated. If the vomiting carries on for more than twenty-four hours, get medical advice. If he is projectile vomiting, contact your doctor immediately as this may be a condition called 'pyloric stenosis' (a narrowing of the part of the stomach that leads to the small intestine). It is more common in boys between two weeks and two months of age and may need surgery to correct it. It could also be a sign of reflux (see above). If sickness is accompanied by diarrhoea, always call a doctor.

Spots and blotches

Milk spots, or milia, are tiny white or yellow bumps which often appear on a new baby's face. Don't be tempted to squeeze them as you may scar the skin or cause an infection. They will disappear within a few weeks.

Babies sometimes get a heat rash – usually a fine pattern of tiny red spots which come and go. It should disappear once the baby's temperature is lowered. Always check that you are not covering your baby in too many layers. Remember that swaddling should be done with a light cotton sheet rather than a blanket. In the summer months make sure your baby is cool and protected from the sun. In really hot weather a nappy, vest and light cotton sheet is enough for him at night.

If your baby has crusty red spots, is bringing up thick curdled milk, is unsettled and not sleeping well he may have a milk allergy. Breastfed babies can get this too – see Eczema above.

Sticky eye

Sticky eye can appear as early as a couple of days after a baby is born. It happens when a tear duct is blocked. A baby's eyelashes stick together when he sleeps and there can be some yellow discharge.

Dip cotton wool in some tepid saline solution (see Colds above

on making your own) and wipe the (closed) eye across the lid –
from his nose towards the ear – at least twice a day. You can also
use breastmilk, which is a great natural antiseptic, as is cooled
chamomile tea. If sticky eye doesn't clear up after a few days, or
if the eye becomes red, see your doctor to make sure it isn't
conjunctivitis, or needs treatment with antibiotic cream.

Teething

Teething pain can start long before outward or obvious signs
of teeth. The symptoms include dribbling, red cheeks, raised
temperature and diarrhoea.

Teething gel is very effective. Once a baby reaches three months
he can have Calpol (liquid Paracetamol). Some parents swear
by homeopathic teething powders which come in pre-measured
sachets and are tipped into your baby's mouth. (One father
claimed this worked because his baby was so stunned by the
sensation of the white granules that he forgot the pain of his
teeth.)

Temperature

A baby's temperature up to the age of six months should be
between 98° and 99°F. If it goes above 100°F try to bring it
down. Sponge your baby with warm water (not tepid as this can
make a baby shiver and his body will react by raising his temperature) and reduce by a layer the amount of clothing he is wearing.
Once your baby is over three months you can give him Calpol.

Encourage him to drink so he does not get dehydrated. If his
temperature continues to rise call for medical advice. If at any
stage a temperature is accompanied by a rash, or if your baby is
floppy, short of breath or refusing fluids, call for medical help
immediately.

If your baby's temperature drops below 95°F he is in danger of being too cold and again this needs medical help. Wrap him in more clothes or a blanket and hold him close to you to warm him up.

The temperature in your baby's bedroom should be between 60° and 70°F.

Thrush

Newborn babies occasionally get oral thrush. White or creamy patches develop inside their mouths and are distinctive because they can't be wiped away. Thrush may be aggravated by teats that haven't been sterilized properly, or can be passed back and forth from a mother's breast. Your doctor can prescribe an anti-fungal cream.

Mums' ailments

'When you're pregnant people fuss over you and ask how you are. Once your baby arrives they ask how he is and forget to ask about you. But you can feel like wet washing put through a mangle and wonder if anyone cares. Be kind to yourself: you will get back to "normal" but don't despair if it takes time. And don't forget to look after yourself as well as your baby. Here are some ideas that might help.'
Barbara

Bleeding

You will bleed after both a vaginal and caesarean delivery, and the blood loss can be very heavy at first – more than for a heavy period – and can last up to six weeks. You can get extra-thick maternity towels (you can even wear more than one at a time), for when sanitary towels aren't enough.

Hot sweats

Women sometimes get hot sweats for a few weeks after giving birth as their hormones settle down. You may wake at night to find your sheets are drenched. Keep a glass of water by the bed as well as a change of night clothes. It's no fun, but it will pass.

Insomnia

Yes, it is possible to be exhausted and yet at the same time be unable to sleep. Many new mums find this and it does pass. In the meantime, use tried and tested remedies such as a warm bath with lavender oil before going to bed or a milky drink. A herbal remedy such as valerian can help bring on sleep but should *not* be used if you are breastfeeding.

Mastitis

Mastitis is exceptionally painful. It happens when the breasts become engorged with milk or a milk duct gets blocked and an infection sets in. It can be accompanied by a temperature and flu-like symptoms and may even need to be treated with antibiotics.

Keep feeding your baby as this will help to drain the breast. If you think he may not be latching on properly get some expert breastfeeding help (see p. 42). Try expressing at the end of feeds to empty your breasts completely. You can also massage your breasts in the bath or place a hot flannel on them to encourage the ducts to unblock.

'The mastitis happened very quickly, within minutes: my breast was like a rock and I had a high temperature. I nearly passed out because I felt so faint. I went downstairs to get my breast pump to express off the milk but felt so ill I couldn't put the pump together. So I sat in the bath trying to massage my breast, sobbing. It felt as if someone had punched me. I can honestly say it was worse than the pain of childbirth. The doctor came and prescribed antibiotics – which fortunately cleared it up very fast.'
Nicola Ripon

Postnatal depression

'Three months after my boys were born I was at a postnatal check-up telling the obstetrician who had delivered them how blissfully happy I was. And I was . . . But as I said my goodbyes she asked if I had anything on my mind. Feeling rather foolish to mention it, I told her I had had a splitting headache every day since the birth and wondered if she might know why.

'I will be for ever grateful to her for recognizing – and telling me kindly and gently – that I was probably suffering from postnatal depression. It had never occurred to me that something as "ordinary" as headaches could have been a symptom. Nor indeed any of the other symptoms like the tiredness, the insomnia, the aching body, the dread I felt at the sound of a baby's cry, my fears about my ability to be a good parent, even the constant tears which I put down to feeling a little emotional. I covered it all up by racing around doing 101 different things and putting on a show of cheerful normality. I even convinced myself!

'I am grateful to my obstetrician because I sought treatment straight away and recovered. I would urge any mum who feels in any way "not quite right" to talk to someone, in case they have postnatal depression. I know how hard it can be to do this because of the stigma attached to depression. I still find it hard to admit I had PND, even though I'm writing about it here. Since I started to talk about it to others I've discovered that loads of other mums have had it too, but didn't like to say.

'It's so wonderful when you get better because you enjoy your baby (in my case babies) so much more. And it's only once you're over it that you truly begin to realize how miserable it was making you.'
Barbara

It may seem strange, but some women can get postnatal depression (PND) and not even know. Some who suffer mildly will recover without ever realizing they had it, and those who get it badly may take months to recognize what they're going through, even though it is very debilitating. Maybe it's the turmoil that mums go through after childbirth that masks the problem. Or maybe new mothers, aware that feeling tearful at this time is normal, turn a blind eye to the signs. The sad thing about this is that postnatal depression that goes undiagnosed and untreated can rob a mother of some of the joy of being with her baby.

Many new mums – around 80 per cent – get the 'baby blues' soon after giving birth. Most recover in a few days. For some though, the baby blues don't disappear. If you are still feeling weepy and 'down' after more than two weeks, it could be PND and you might want to think about getting help.

There is another form of PND which doesn't start out as the

baby blues. This depression develops more slowly, and can appear at any time in the first year after the birth. The fact that it can manifest itself so late may be why mothers don't always recognize the symptoms. So how can you spot it, or how could you miss it?

The trouble with PND is that many of its symptoms may not immediately strike you as being signs of depression. You might – understandably – confuse them with the demands of having a baby: severe fatigue, lethargy, irritability, tension, anxiety, insomnia and weepiness. Some women report having severe pains in their back, chest, neck or head.

Other, perhaps more obvious signs of depression include: panic attacks, feelings of worthlessness, insecurity, worry about the future, not wanting to leave the house or meet friends, low self-esteem, an inability to concentrate, and being unable to cope, including with a crying baby. In severe cases there may be obsessive thoughts, including suicidal ones.

If you read up about PND you'll find that most estimates of the numbers of mothers who get it are between 10 and 15 per cent, but it could well be more. The magazine *Prima Baby* conducted a survey among its readers and concluded that nearly one in five mothers may experience postnatal depression. Thirty per cent of women who suffer from PND are thought to be still suffering by the time of their child's first birthday.

This moving testimony was written (anonymously) to demonstrate how easy it can be to miss the symptoms, and how debilitating PND can be if not treated.

> *'After my boys were born I felt physically unwell with insomnia, backache and an unshakeable debilitating exhaustion. All symptoms could have been attributed to carrying twins followed by having a caesarean section. However the diagnosis didn't feel right.*
>
> *'Six months on I felt no better. I wasn't really enjoying*

the babies even in peaceful moments and I couldn't get myself to do anything. Every task seemed a chore and the list of chores seemed endless. Lack of parental joy and the niggling fear that I was missing the innate maternal instinct others seemed to have, resulted in my guilt. My guilt was then compounded by the fact that I felt I should be happy but wasn't. What was wrong with me?

'It took time, but it finally dawned on me that I had postnatal depression. What else could explain feeling empty when looking at my two boys when everyone else melted at the sight of four blue eyes peering at them? And I couldn't remember when the last time was that I laughed. Or smiled. Or felt anything other than heavy pressing responsibility to just do and do and do.

'PND is so easy to mask to the rest of the world. People would often comment on how amazing it was that I was coping but they only saw me at my best: outdoors in the fresh air, pushing a buggy holding two rosy-cheeked infants. The reality was that I had no choice. Life expects too much to just fold back one's arms and let infants cry. And I didn't want to admit to anyone what was wrong because I felt there was something wrong with me, the stigma of any form of depression.

'It's taken me nearly three years to get over it. It was overnight – one morning I woke up and it was gone. Now there is only the regret to live with. All that time lost . . .

'With hindsight I wish I had had an official diagnosis, and therapy and/or drugs. I did nothing. The added advantage of having a diagnosis – assuming you have a sensitive doctor – is that by explaining PND in medical terms it may make it easier for your husband to understand that there really is something wrong with you – which will also reassure him that this very difficult situation will eventually end.

'Of tremendous help is to speak to others in the same situation. The reassurance, even to yourself, that you are not "mad", that you are not a "bad mum", and that you are not alone, is priceless.'
'Melanie'

Treatment for mild PND may be a course of counselling but for more severe cases drugs are usually offered and have to be taken for several months. Unfortunately women sometimes have to self-diagnose: there are stories of doctors not only failing to look for signs of PND in mothers who are clearly at high risk, but also of failing to notice the symptoms even when they are blindingly obvious. (Some women are known to be more at risk. These include: mothers of multiples, women with a previous history of depression, women with relationship problems or those who have had a difficult birth or have had IVF, to name but some examples.)

You might have some success in relieving your symptoms, particularly the fatigue or insomnia, with alternative therapies such as acupuncture. Cranial osteopathy may also be helpful (see under Colic).

It's also really important to rest as much as you can; tiredness can exacerbate the problem. Some recent Australian research showed that mothers who learned to manage sleep problems with their babies were less likely to suffer from PND.

Post-partum tummy and getting back into shape

Please don't beat yourself up if you can't squeeze into your pre-pregnancy clothes as soon as you would like. You can't expect the work of nine months to disappear in a flash – set yourself a goal of nine months to get back to the way you were, and if you get there before then, hooray!

Hospital physiotherapists should show you some gentle post-natal exercises you can work on almost immediately after the birth. Most mums though, especially first-timers, are too exhausted and overwhelmed to find time or energy to stick to doing them regularly, at least at the beginning.

To be on the safe side (and especially if you have had a caesarean) you shouldn't start a full exercise programme until you have been given the all-clear at your six-week check-up. If you can find a way of getting to a few classes, Pilates is a great shape-restorer. It works on the muscles – the transverse abdominals – that are stretched in pregnancy, and on the pelvic floor, which undergoes trauma during a vaginal birth as well as during your pregnancy (so shouldn't be overlooked if you have a caesarean). For a small number of women that trauma can lead to stress incontinence ('leaking' when you run, cough or sneeze) so the exercises are really worth doing. Once you are familiar with them, practising even just the pelvic floor ones regularly at home – or anywhere you find yourself with a spare moment – will get the muscles back into shape more quickly.

If you haven't got time to do any more than this, don't overlook the fact that carrying a baby round and going out with a pushchair is exercise in itself. Ignore the film stars and models who seem to shrink effortlessly – they too have to work to get there, and probably hire a personal trainer to help them.

Sore nipples

Apart from a strange tingling sensation which some mums get at the beginning of a feed, it should never hurt when you breastfeed (unless you have exceptionally sensitive nipples). On the contrary, it should be a wonderful experience. If your nipples are sore, make sure you are positioning the baby on the breast properly and that he is not sucking for longer than he needs. The first ten days are usually the hardest: try, if you can, to persevere and you should find that you have not only passed the worst of it but that it becomes a real pleasure.

If you find that one breast is more sore than the other, leave it for two feeds to give it a chance to heal. Breastmilk is a great healer as is the air. Grated carrot or cabbage leaves placed in your bra can ease the discomfort, and if you use breast pads change them regularly so your nipples stay dry.

Stitches

These can be uncomfortable for a while and urinating can be difficult. Try pouring a jug of warm water over your stitches when you are on the loo, or urinate in the bath.

You could add some rock salt to your bath water to act as an antiseptic and use a hairdryer on your stitches afterwards to make sure they are really dry. A shower head can be useful for cleaning them.

Vaseline can prevent stitches from drying out and pinching. If you are in a lot of discomfort wrap a bag of frozen peas in a towel and hold it on the spot for ten to fifteen seconds. It might help to sit on a rubber ring for a few days.

Caesarean stitches will dissolve over time, or you may have staples which need to be removed a few days after the operation. Try applying a little pure vitamin E oil on the wound to help soften the skin and minimize scarring as it heals. If the wound starts to gape use some steri-strips (from pharmacies) to hold it back together until you can talk to your midwife.

Stretch marks

There are many creams and oils on the market that can be applied during pregnancy and may prevent stretch marks – but equally may not. Vitamin E cream, applied before and after the birth, is a good bet.

If stretch marks do appear though, it's unlikely they'll go away, but they *will* fade over time. Be careful not to expose them to sunlight as they may burn more readily.

'I was so lucky – despite carrying twins I never got stretch marks. But I was shocked at how dry my skin was after the birth: it was like crêpe paper and was really sensitive when touched. I thought it would never be the same again. In fact it didn't take as long as I feared (a matter of a few weeks). I swear that this oil-based formula with aromatherapy oils – which you can make up at home – did the trick for me:

- 30 ml almond oil
- 15 ml wheatgerm oil
- 10 drops borage seed oil/evening primrose oil
- 5 drops carrot oil
- 7 drops rose oil (Bulgar or Maroc)
- 6 drops lavender oil
- 5 drops tangerine or mandarin oil

'Rub a small amount into the skin twice a day. Cover any areas that have been affected, including tummy, thighs and buttocks.

'Everything I read about the aromatherapy oils recommended here suggested that they were among the few that are widely considered to be safe in pregnancy, so you could think about applying the oil as a preventative measure while you are pregnant. I did, right from the beginning of my pregnancy, and am convinced it helped.

'But if, understandably, you are at all concerned about

using aromatherapy oils when pregnant you could consult
an aromatherapy practitioner, or err on the side of caution
by using a mix of only the vegetable base oils – almond,
wheatgerm, borage seed and carrot – until after your baby
is born, and then adding the rest.'
Barbara

Swollen ankles

Your ankles may continue to be swollen for a while after giving
birth so you need to wear those hideous stockings to keep the
circulation going and prevent clotting. It may feel like the last
straw when you're already struggling to look half-decent, but they
are essential and you won't have to wear them for long. Try
keeping your feet raised whenever you sit down. Some women
swear by drinking herbal teas – fennel or nettle – for reducing
the swelling.

12.

Twin Secrets

There are two things in life for which we are never fully prepared . . . and that is twins.

Josh Billings, nineteenth-century American humorist

'The day my boys were born found me in a state of total *un*preparedness: I hadn't even put up a cot, let alone two, as I was blissfully unaware that caring for two small babies would leave so little time to do anything other than eat and sleep.

'A bit of forethought and planning might have braced me for what lay ahead: one of the most gruelling and exhausting experiences of my life, but also one of the most rewarding. When you're expecting twins, I now know, being prepared is not a luxury, it's a necessity. I also know that twin parents are often as unprepared as I was.

'It has been one of the greatest joys I've known. I just wish I had known a little bit more about what was involved before I started.'
Barbara

'That's where I hope this chapter can help you, with its ideas on getting ready for a double arrival, as well as on using the routines and night-time techniques once your babies are with you, and getting them to work for you. Routine and sleep are the key to moving from the exhausting times to the rewarding ones, as you will find out.

'The advice here is designed to be read in conjunction with the rest of the book – which applies to all babies equally, twins or not. It's meant to be as realistic as possible about some of the challenges you will face, while remaining optimistic that you'll agree that having twins is special.'

Jo

Please note that the references throughout this chapter are mainly to twins. The advice and sentiments apply (almost) equally to triplets, though it will not surprise anyone to know that triplets come with their own unique demands and needs, not all of which can be covered here.

Preparation

Getting used to the news

Being told you have more than one baby on the way is nearly always a shock. For some, the shock soon gives way to excitement at the idea of an 'instant family' (if this is a first pregnancy), the novelty (only one in seventy births is a multiple birth), or the knowledge that having twins can be tremendous fun (which it can). For others, the initial shock gives way to weeks or months of anxiety and uncertainty. It is hardly surprising: a multiple birth means the prospect of a high-risk pregnancy, the possibility of producing low-birthweight babies needing special care, and increased financial and emotional pressures.

Not everyone has a burning desire to be a twin or triplet parent. If you didn't whoop with joy or crack open the champagne when you heard the news, or if you still have serious reservations about what lies ahead, please don't panic. You are not alone.

'It was truly a terrible day when I found out I was having twins. Josh and I had both thought we only wanted one child and we already had him: only in a moment of weakness did Josh agree that it would be nice for him to have a sibling . . . and suddenly I was pregnant!

'It never occurred to me in a million years that there could be more than one baby. I even joked to the ultrasound technician at my scan how awful it would be to check the "more than one foetus" box. A minute later she was saying, "You know what we were just joking about? Well there are two in there."

'I started crying and Josh went grey.

'Now, call me crazy but I think the medical community should seriously consider offering counselling after dropping that news on you. I know it is easy news compared to what many people discover at scans, but it was life-changing for us. I resented the fact that someone had changed the rules without consulting me, and I no longer felt in control.

'The weirdest thing was that every person we told either said what wonderful news it was or just laughed. No one was any help and we became more and more overwhelmed by the whole thing. Whenever we thought about how we were going to cope we felt sick.

'Judging by most people's reaction when I tell them this, I'm not the only one to have felt this way: maybe I'm just more open about it. I have never felt obliged to lie so I don't offend people: I have always managed to separate the love and responsibility I have felt for each of my children from the overwhelming burden and disruption that having twins was to our life plan.'

Jacki

As you come to terms with your news, others will be full of well-meaning comments: having twins makes parents public property, open to intrusive (and not necessarily constructive) observations such as 'Do twins run in your family?', 'Were they conceived naturally?', 'You poor thing . . .' (especially with triplets) and of course, 'Double trouble!' A sense of humour or a thick skin is probably the best antidote. View this as preparation for what is to come, which is star status/unwanted attention (depending on your viewpoint) every time you step outside the front door.

If you didn't know that there is a network of twins clubs, now may be the time to investigate. Some are more active than others, organizing coffee mornings for expectant mums, running toddler groups and second-hand sales, and producing regular newsletters. Others are simply a point of contact between parents of multiples. Either way, even someone who is not a natural 'joiner' may find their local club a wonderful resource. No matter how many other people offer you advice, unless they have had twins they will never know what it feels like to be the mother of two tiny creatures at once.

You might want to join Tamba, the Twins and Multiple Births Association, to access information. Tamba runs a confidential telephone listening and information service called Twinline (see Notes, p. 290) for parents or parents-to-be.

Whether your hospital offers specialist antenatal classes is down to the luck of the draw. If yours does, don't leave it too late to attend as 50 per cent of twins arrive before thirty-seven weeks, which is considered gestation for twins (thirty-four weeks for triplets), and many parents are caught unawares. (Gestation for a single baby is forty weeks.)

The Multiple Births Foundation runs regular evening sessions on 'Preparing for Twins or Triplets' in London and these are open to anyone who can get to them (check their website for details).

Equipment

'Do I really need two of everything?' is an often-heard cry. Unfortunately, there are few economies of scale with twins or triplets. Here's where buying second-hand can come in. Your local twins club may have a sale of used clothes and equipment or may be able to put you in touch with a mum who is keen to sell her baby items.

You'll need two (or three) of most of the items listed in chapter 1, in particular two rocker chairs and double the number of bottles. You may need only one (large) activity mat, and if your babies are going to sleep in the same room one cot mobile is enough (or the competing tinkles will fray your nerves), as is one Slumber Bear/lullaby soother (unless the cots are a long way apart). Bypass moses baskets and put your babies straight into a cot together (swaddled); they can stay together for several months. (Recent research has concluded that it *is* safe for babies to share a cot.)

Other items specifically for twins or triplets and which you might find useful are a twin nursing pillow and a hands-free bottle-feeding system (see Notes, p. 290 for where to buy). There is a twin baby-carrier on the market, but carrying two babies at a time may not suit everyone.

'A few months after my twins were born I took over the running of the Central London Twins Club and have since met many twin mums and mums-to-be. I've been amazed how often the same question comes up: time and again everyone wants to know which is the best buggy to buy. It comes before questions on feeding, sleeping and routines, which is why there's a little more detail here on buggies than for other equipment.'
Barbara

The truth is that there is no ideal pushchair, but there may be an ideal one for you, so doing research before buying this essential and expensive piece of equipment is important. A quick way to do that research could be to pop the question to members of your twins club. You will soon know all you ever wanted to – and more. It's a hot topic – and almost as personal a choice as buying a car.

Buying a buggy (as they are often called) for twins is not as straightforward as buying one for a single baby, where one good-quality pushchair can serve from birth to toddlerhood. A high-quality, sturdy, double pushchair starts quite heavy and becomes heavier as your babies put on weight. A lightweight pushchair is an obvious alternative, but it may not be sturdy enough to accommodate bigger babies. Then there's the choice between three wheels and four. The general view is that whichever you choose, swivel front wheels are essential. Oddly, three-wheelers are usually wider than four-wheelers, and although they are usually easier to manoeuvre, they can be harder to collapse and put in a car.

You may also need single buggies so you can take your babies out separately. (You can buy stroller connectors to clip two together if you need to, though this is not recommended except for short journeys on reasonably flat terrain.) In short, when it comes to buggies you may have to face buying more than one.

> '*Measure your doorway, consider whether you will be going up and down a lot of stairs (lightweight would be important), are you getting in and out of the car a lot (easy folding a must), where will it be stored in the house (how big is it when folded), are you mainly taking it to the park (big wheels), or in and out of shops (width, easy turning, good storage basket)? And if your answer is yes to all of these, what is most important to you?*'
> **Susan**

'My advice is buy your first buggy second-hand because you'll only use it for eight or nine months and then invest in a high-quality lightweight umbrella fold.'
Kate

'The mountain buggy is my favourite:
- It is strong and has big pneumatic wheels which makes the ride much smoother
- It is great for rough terrain (some car parks, country walks, etc.)
- It is very easy to put up and fold down — almost one-handed
- It is very comfy
- It has a good basket underneath for shopping
- It is a bit heavy due to size but not unmanageable.

Cost is about £600 but the buggy lasts for ever and takes the children until they are about four or five if necessary.'
Dan

'We bought the Graco Duo Sport which after twenty-one months is a bit bent at the front (from being lifted on and off buses) but still going strong. One reason we got it was that it is narrower than the trendy three-wheelers.'
Ann

'The In-step Twin Nipper is the best thing that we have bought for our twins — I think it is the lightest and narrowest buggy on the market yet it is very manoeuvrable — we love it.'
Penny

'The Maclaren Twin Traveller is great, used from birth as the seats go back all the way. Still useful when walking and when the boys nap — they are fourteen and a half months now and it is still going strong.'
Sherry

'I wouldn't touch Maclaren. We've had three double buggies and they all let us down.'
Laura

'The Mamas and Papas lightweight Twin Aria was great when the boys were small and is still useful for getting round the shops. But it's no good for long walks now (small wheels) so we use the three-wheeler XTS Twin Twister which is fabulous. Easy to push and to fold.'
Brenda

Whether it's buggies or rocker chairs, however, don't leave the preparations too late. It's not a great idea to be hunting for equipment with two or more small babies in tow.

Planning some extra help

'As parents of twins, two babies means that no matter how hard you try to stay on top of the laundry, bottles, cleaning, grocery shopping, nappy changing, etc. it will never be enough because you're shorthanded. Lower expectations, get as much help as you can, say yes to all offers of help and most important be kind to each other, it will get easier in time.'
Angie

'Is it really that much harder having two babies than just one?'
A man

There's no getting away from it: having more than one baby is a lot more work so think ahead about roping in any help you can. Many expectant twin parents make the mistake of assuming they will manage without help, but often struggle. (Triplet parents usually know that they need help; it often comes as a surprise to learn that there is no free state help available for either triplet or twin families.) Whatever support you can find – whether it is from family, friends or paid help – take it.

If you are relying on friends, don't allow their promises to turn hollow. Plan lists of things to be done so that when they turn up, they will not be tempted just to sit and chat. Try asking them how much time they can offer and tell them what will need doing. To avoid being the one who makes endless cups of tea for visitors, stick notices on cupboard doors indicating where the tea, coffee, sugar and mugs are. Keeping a copy of your routine in a prominent place will enable everyone to see at a glance what is happening and when.

Don't be embarrassed about leaning on friends when you have twins or triplets. And don't feel awkward if what you want them to do is shop, cook or even clean. You might find some prefer ironing or hoovering to changing nappies – or even to making conversation with a distracted new mum.

Be aware that grandparents, if they are around, may be daunted by the prospect of helping out with two babies, but be reluctant to admit it. You could ask if they would be prepared to take one baby for a few hours now and again so you can have some one-to-one time with the other.

Students studying for childcare qualifications are sometimes available to help parents of multiples for free as they need to gain practical experience on their courses. CACHE, the body responsible for childcare training standards, has information on which colleges place students in families. The placements are arranged in advance so you will need to look into this well ahead of time.

Home Start is a voluntary organization which helps families in need of support. The help is free but amounts only to a few hours per week and again you should enquire well in advance. You may also discover other voluntary organizations able to offer help in your local community.

If you can afford paid help but are not sure if it's a valuable way to spend money, think again: it is. You are about to face stresses and strains that are hard to imagine beforehand. Any back-up in caring for your babies, or helping around the house, will pay dividends. If some paid cleaning help conserves your energy when you need it most, you will be investing in your own and your babies' well-being.

Other options for paid help – au pairs, mother's helps, doulas, nannies, night nannies and maternity nurses – are covered in chapter 13. At the upper end of the scale (both experience- and cost-wise) is the maternity nurse, who can be a life-saver with twins, not just in establishing routines and sleep, but could be invaluable in helping new parents cope with what are very often small, premature babies. A cheaper option might be a maternity trainee, or a maternity nanny, who will do days only (see p. 263). One triplet mum even paid a trainee midwife, whom she met while in hospital, to help her for a few days when she and her babies returned home. Some parents find they can cope if they have an occasional night's sleep and will book a night nanny to help out now and then.

One word of warning however: don't fall into the trap of thinking that qualified childcare is the best or only option, even with low-birthweight babies. Since maternity nurses and nannies rarely offer to help with household chores and expect you to feed them while they are with you, they have their drawbacks. The key is to work out what type of help, in the broadest sense, will be most useful in your particular situation – family and financial.

Once your babies have arrived

Low-birthweight babies are sometimes jaundiced and need to be placed under a light source. They may also have low blood-sugar levels. In this case a doctor will recommend feeding them formula milk but make sure that you understand, and are happy with, any such medical advice.

Hospitals are not allowed to recommend one baby formula over another. You will be asked what you prefer – which you might find strange if you haven't given this question any thought.

Babies in special care

Your babies, or possibly just one of them, may need to go into special care; 50 per cent of multiples spend some time in a special care unit. It may seem a daunting prospect, but a visit beforehand to the SCBU (Special Care Baby Unit) is a good way of preparing yourself for this eventuality. (The care for premature singletons is the same as for twins but since the likelihood of a premature birth is greater with multiples the advice has been included in this chapter.)

> 'It helped me tremendously. Seeing the incubators, the endless wires, the bleeping monitors, the frequently sounding alarms and the frighteningly small babies does wonders to objectively shock the system without the raw emotion attached when that child is your own. When the girls arrived early and went into intensive care I felt secure

when I first saw them. I knew that both they and all the attached apparatus were "normal". Knowledge lends confidence and nothing is needed more than reassurance in those first hours.'
Mindy

You could ask if the unit will help you do 'kangaroo care', where babies are placed close to your skin inside your clothes. This is not only comforting for a baby but also stimulates the mother's milk supply.

Establishing your breastfeeding early should be possible even if your babies are born prematurely. Start as soon as you can. You will need a breast pump (preferably an electric one – see p. 286 on hiring or buying one). Hospitals have breast pumps but they are often industrial-looking and unwieldy. (Until your milk comes in you are advised to express your colostrum by hand as this is known to help in the long-term success of breastfeeding.) It's wise to express three-hourly and avoid gaps of more than four hours during the day. You could also express in the middle of the night, if you can face it. A photo of your baby/babies, or sitting by the incubator, may stimulate your milk flow. Breastmilk will keep for twenty-four hours in a fridge and can be frozen for up to three months. Thawed milk can be kept in the fridge for up to twelve hours.

If you can't breastfeed, your babies will probably be offered a formula designed for low-birthweight and premature babies – Nutriprem. This is given only on the advice of doctors and needs to be prescribed if it is to be continued once you get home. If you are not offered Nutriprem, you may like to enquire about it. (Some mothers report that their babies become constipated on Nutriprem as a result of its high iron content. If this happens, talk to your doctor.) Small babies need latex rather than silicone teats to ease sucking, and the hospital will provide these.

This can be a very stressful time for a new mum. Travelling to and from the hospital is hard enough without the worries you may have about your babies' health. Returning home without your babies, or returning with one and not the other, can be a surreal experience. In some cases hospitals don't have enough special care beds for a set of twins or triplets and you may need to be transferred to another one. In the worst instance your babies could be separated and sent to different hospitals and, although this is not likely, it can and does happen and is worth being prepared for.

Special care can also lull you into a false sense of comfort about the task of caring for two babies and you may be taken aback when you finally go it alone. Think about getting a friend or relative to be with you when you first get home.

Can I breastfeed twins?

It is sometimes assumed, whether by midwives, maternity nurses or health visitors, that twin mums either can't or won't breastfeed and all-too-often this becomes a self-fulfilling prophecy. If you really want to breastfed your twins, there is every reason to believe you will be able to. Your success might depend on the confidence and support you get from those around you.

> 'I breastfed my twins exclusively for three months (they were born weighing 6lb), and then mixed-fed until they were about eight months, gradually changing over about one feed a month.
>
> 'I was lucky to be on the one-to-one scheme with the midwife – she got me off to a good start. People always assume that with twins you don't breastfeed, so when I told her I wanted to she was delighted and encouraged me, explaining that my body would respond to meet demand.

She instilled confidence in me from early in my pregnancy, so by the time they were born it didn't even occur to me not to breastfeed. I had a c-section, and as soon as we were in the recovery room she got them to latch on.

'Personally I found breastfeeding much easier – once we'd all three got the hang of it, it was the most relaxing part of my day; it meant I had my hands free while feeding – and the idea of sterilizing and preparing formula for two babies from day one was a real disincentive.

'I was lucky: I was overflowing with milk and my babies fed well, and I had a midwife who gave me the confidence I could do it.'
Jo K

If you are determined to breastfeed your twins but find they struggle to latch on, you could seek out specialist breastfeeding help. It is best not to try feeding them together until any problems are overcome and your breastfeeding is going smoothly. Small babies often need to put on weight before they can latch on readily; they may also find it hard to suck for long enough to get a full feed. One option in both these situations is to give your babies expressed breastmilk from a bottle. Use latex teats (see above).

You may be told by your midwife that if you resort to using a bottle (even of expressed breastmilk) your babies may refuse to breastfeed. Please consider two things before taking heed of this advice: first, it is extremely important that your babies get their milk *somehow* or they will start to lose weight; second, it is by no means a foregone conclusion that a baby offered a bottle subsequently refuses the breast (see p. 52 on nipple/teat confusion). Try to offer the breast for a few minutes at the beginning of each feed before offering the bottle so your babies come to associate the breast with feeding. When you offer the bottle, run the teat over your babies' lips in order to encourage them to open their mouths for their milk, which they need to do in order to breastfeed. Do this in preference to pushing the bottle straight into their mouths, which can make them lazy.

Midwives sometimes suggest cup-feeding a baby in order to reduce the risk of a baby becoming attached to the bottle, but some mums find that sitting a tiny baby up and feeding him from a cup is quite disheartening. Don't follow this advice if it makes you feel uncomfortable.

However, if you can't breastfeed your twins or if you decide that you don't want to, for whatever reason, don't beat yourself up about it. It is not at all uncommon for twin mums to find themselves in either of these situations, as you will discover if you talk to other twin parents. Breastfeeding two babies requires a lot of effort on the part of your body and you may not feel up to it. You can only do what works best for you. One thing that may work well is to use formula in addition to breastfeeding. This is known as mixed feeding or 'topping up'.

How to get twins into a feeding routine

> 'My health visitor told me it was impossible to get twins into a routine. Thank goodness we proved her wrong.'
> **Mindy**

It certainly *is* possible to get twins into a routine, even if it takes a little longer to get things running smoothly than it does with a single baby. There is no magic formula involved: when you are ready, you choose a routine to suit your babies' age and weight and work towards feeding both at the same time, as soon as you and they are able to do so.

You should start a log charting both babies' feeding and sleeping patterns as soon as you can. This will help you work out when they need their naps and which routine will suit them best. Logs have the added benefit of helping you to chart your babies' progress, which might seem elusive on a day-to-day basis.

Feeding two babies at once is something of an art, whether on the breast or with bottles. You don't have to do this, and some parents either don't want to or find it doesn't work for them, but if you do, it will make the routines easier to follow. It may also be the only way you can snatch some time between feeds to do anything else. A second pair of hands always helps, but if you are on your own for most of the time do persevere. With some trial and error you will find a way through. Here are some ideas on how you might feed two at the same time.

Before you start, you will need to wake your babies one after the other. If they are both sleepy you might want to wake one, take off any blankets or sheets and leave him to come round while you wake the other baby. Then return to the first, change his nappy, and do the same for the second. Do this at the start of each day too.

Breastfeeding two babies together takes time to master and is best left until your breastfeeding is established with both babies latching on and sucking well. Once you feel you are ready to 'tandem feed', sit in a comfortable chair with your back well supported and with plenty of pillows or cushions. You need to be within reach of your babies if you have no one to hand them to you. When you first try this, make sure someone is around to help get your babies positioned comfortably and then eased off at the end of the feed. Use pillows or cushions to support them or try a v-shaped pillow or specialist twin feeding pillow.

The 'rugby tackle' hold is popular: position your babies with their heads almost touching each other and their legs under your arms. Have your phone within reach if you think you will need to take calls and have a glass of water or juice near you: breastfeeding two babies means eating and drinking vast quantities. If you are all well supported you should be able to wind the first baby to finish while the other is still drinking.

> '*I did both of them at the same time: I would sit on the sofa with one baby on each side of me, get my v-shaped pillow out, then put one baby in place in the "rugby-tackle" position, then the other. One would generally finish earlier so I could burp him/her while the other one carried on feeding. When feeding in the bedroom I had a good chair next to the bed with wide arms that would support the v-cushion. I would lie them both on the bed in front of me and then latch one on, then the other. The key was to have a comfortable position for feeding which supported my back. Sitting in bed was no good.*
>
> '*At night I was led by whoever woke first – I would start that one off, and my husband would gently wake the second one and bring that one to me. He (and often I) would then doze while they fed and he would then put the one who finished first back to bed, before returning to sleep himself. Having another pair of hands at night was very helpful as well as being good moral support.*'
>
> **Jo K**

The downside to tandem-feeding for some mothers is that they never get any one-to-one feeding time with their babies. No one can really understand these dilemmas unless they have fed twins themselves so you might want to talk to someone in your twins club who has been through the experience.

Low-birthweight babies need to be fed separately, particularly if you are breastfeeding, until they gain weight and are feeding confidently. This can leave you feeling as if you are feeding, winding and changing without respite. It will get easier.

If you are bottle-feeding you may still find that small babies need to be held and fed separately for a while. Once your babies are strong enough you can put them in their rocker chairs (some people use their portable car seats), sit between them with your back supported, and hold the bottles in their mouths. If you feel uncomfortable feeding your babies without any physical contact, you could try placing both on your lap, supported on pillows, and bottle-feed them together. An alternative is to put two pillows on the sofa in front of you, place one baby on each and sitting in front of the sofa feed both at the same time.

Mixed-feeding a combination of breast and formula milk (or 'topping up') is popular with twin mums; mums of singletons sometimes do this too. If you have someone to help, you can breastfeed one baby while your helper bottle-feeds the other. At the next feed swap over. An alternative is to feed one baby on the breast for half a feed (maybe limiting his time to around fifteen minutes) before moving straight to the next baby, while your helper tops the first baby up with half a bottle-feed.

If you are mixed-feeding and have no one to help, you could – once your babies are sucking well – put one baby in a rocker chair in front of you, settle the other on the breast and use a spare hand to give a bottle to the baby in the chair. Another option is to try a hands-free bottle.

The hardest part of feeding two babies at once can be when you have to stop feeding both babies in order to wind one. You might need to develop your own hands-free system. Some bottle-feeding mums find that once their babies are a few weeks old (and if born prematurely are past the 8lb mark when their necks will have strengthened and their suck will be stronger), they can carefully wedge a towel or muslin under the bottle of a baby sitting in a rocker chair for a couple of minutes so that he can continue to feed while the other one is winded. If you do this, keep your baby within arm's reach at all times and under no circumstances leave him unattended.

Don't be afraid to resort to using a dummy if this helps keep the peace. The bottom line is: do what feels right for all of you. These are suggestions that work for many twin mums.

Which routine should I follow?

Follow the routine you would choose for a single baby. If your babies are small (less than 7lb) you would normally start by feeding them two-and-a-half-hourly during the day until they reach the 7lb mark. But if you are on your own for most of the time this will mean a lot of work for you so start your twins on the three-hourly routine. You will need to feed small babies three-hourly during the night until they are about 6lb; then wait until they wake naturally. Don't stretch them to sleep longer until they reach 7lb. This can be hard going while it lasts, but it will get easier.

If your babies have been in special care they will probably be on a three-hourly (round-the-clock) routine which you can continue. Again, don't stretch their feeds or sleep until they reach 7lb.

Some twins may even leave special care on a four-hourly feeding routine, which you can also continue, but if you feel it is pushing them too hard (maybe they are not sleeping a long stretch at night as soon as you might hope, or maybe you are having trouble keeping them going between feeds) try a routine which feeds a little more frequently until you feel your babies are ready to be stretched, such as the three- or three-and-a-half-hourly routines. You will not be taking a step backwards if you do this; in fact you will probably be saving yourself trouble later down the line. Many premature babies are very sleepy in the first few weeks and it is not difficult to stretch them to feed every four hours. However, after a few weeks they will wake up, be more active and get very hungry, and four-hourly feeding at this stage is often not enough, unless they are fed four-hourly round-the-clock. If you want to stretch them to sleep longer at night they will have to be fed more frequently during the day or they will not be getting all the milk they need.

Parents of small babies are sometimes lulled into a sense of security: their baby/babies sleep much of the day and do not need frequent feeding. Then, when they become more alert and demand to be fed more often, the parents feel that things are going backwards and are reluctant to change the pattern they are in. You should not see this as a backwards step, but more as an adaptation to your baby's changing needs and one which will be temporary.

How do I comfort two babies when they cry?

Babies cry. That is a fact of life and doesn't mean you are a bad parent. When you have two babies crying it can be very stressful. Remind yourself that you can really only comfort one at a time, and don't allow yourself to feel guilty or inadequate. Your babies will suffer no psychological damage. Life with twins will place many unique demands on you but also bring many unique rewards. Try looking at this as one of the demands that is balanced out by the rewards.

If you are feeding your babies separately you may confront this problem frequently as one baby waits impatiently for his milk but cannot be attended to. Having him in his rocker chair in front of you so you can talk to him while you are feeding his twin might help, as might a dummy.

Night-time

Getting your twins to sleep through the night will be your life-saver. All the techniques are in chapter 9, but here are some thoughts on how to follow them with two babies.

Start with the bedtime ritual (p. 94), taking each stage with both babies at the same time, or as closely as you can achieve this. This ritual is such an important part of helping your babies to sleep well that it's worth viewing it as one of the most precious parts of the day and being rigorous about not letting it slip. A second pair of hands will always make this easier but if you are putting your babies to bed on your own here is some guidance:

Prepare the bath (either a baby bath or your big bath with a baby support) and lay out two changing mats, towels and nappies, two sets of night clothes and the massage cream. Take your babies into the bathroom and lay them on the changing mats on the floor (or place one on a changing mat and the other in a rocker chair). Undress one and bath him. Dry him and either keep him swaddled in his towel while you then bath the other, or dress him, lie him safely on the mat, towel or in a rocker chair, and repeat the whole process with your other baby. Once they are about four weeks old you could massage both, even if briefly, before putting on their night clothes.

Following all these steps in one place means you never leave a baby out of your sight or in the bath unattended. In time, and once you have progressed to bathing them in the big bath, it will become easier to do both babies at once.

You don't have to bath both babies every day. In the first few weeks you can top 'n' tail them, or alternate them so that one is bathed and one is top 'n' tailed each day.

Take your babies into the bedroom, keep the lights low and feed them, preferably together or one after the other, depending on what is working best for you. If one finishes sooner, pop him in a rocker chair while he waits; you can then put both babies down to sleep at the same time. Now follow the techniques in chapter 9.

When it comes to the dream feed, you may find it easier to feed one baby first and then wake the other, but again it will save time if you can do both at once (you will probably be anxious to get to bed).

To set a base time for the night-time feeds, be guided by whichever baby needs to be fed soonest. When you have calculated that base time use it for both, waking the second baby at the same time (if he is not already awake) and feeding them together if you can.

If you are not feeding your babies together, you need to feed them straight after each other, as you would during the day, even if it means waking one. If the second one is awake and gets impatient to be fed, keep a dummy handy.

As you follow the night-time guidelines on settling an unsettled baby or on stretching night-time sleep, use spaced soothing as you would with one baby. Most twins do not wake from the sounds of the other, as long as they have shared a room from the start. When you go to soothe one, it's unlikely that your doing so will wake his twin.

You will have read in chapter 9 that it can be hard-going for you during the first few days of teaching a baby to sleep. This is particularly true with twins, but the reward of having two babies sleep through the night usually gives twin parents extra determination to see it through.

> '*I already had a set of twins aged three and a half when my second set arrived. The older ones had been demand-fed and slept where they seemed happiest — usually downstairs in their rocker chairs. I spent many nights on the floor next to them as I was getting up so often there was no point going to bed. To get them to fall asleep they were rocked, pushed in the pushchair or taken out in baby carriers. Late at night my husband and I could be seen walking up and down the high street trying to calm them.*
>
> '*On the rare occasions I ventured out during the day,*

the babies would start screaming for a feed (even though they had been fed an hour before) and I would run home as fast as I could, close to tears, and angry about the comments people had made about the babies crying.

'At around a year they eventually started to sleep for most of the night, but even at the age of three and a half they were still waking early in the morning and refusing to settle. So when I had twins again I asked Jo to help me get them into a routine as I couldn't bear the thought of four children keeping us awake for years to come and turning our lives into chaos.

'When Sofia and Cara were two weeks old and had put on some weight (were over 7lb) they were put on a three-hourly routine. It was fantastic because by planning ahead I could get out of the house without having to race back within minutes.

'I breastfed them with formula top-ups at each feed, always starting with the smallest baby as she was too tired after a bottle to latch on. They had formula at night. It took just over a week for them to settle after the 7 p.m. feed and sleep through until 11 p.m. This meant I could get my older two ready for bed, make dinner and enjoy time with my husband instead of running up and down stairs all night or walking the streets with wailing babies.

'At the beginning the girls would wake at around 3 a.m. and over the weeks their feeds were stretched: after two weeks they weren't waking until 4.30. We would still have to go in between six and 6.30 when I would give them a reduced feed. When the babies were eight weeks old they started to sleep from 11 p.m. to 7 a.m. Four weeks later I dropped the 11 p.m. dream feed and they slept from seven to seven. I never ever, in my wildest dreams, thought I would be able to say "my twins sleep through the night".'

Kate

Where do they sleep and when do I separate them?

Some parents of twins remark that their babies seem happier if they're allowed to sleep together, re-creating the closeness they shared in the womb. Start by putting them side to side at the end of the cot (feet to end). When they get bigger and begin to wriggle, place them side by side crossways in the middle of the cot, and when their arms or legs start straying put one at each end of the cot, head in the middle, feet to end.

You will know when it's finally time to separate them: they will wriggle so much they will wake each other, either after a few weeks or possibly as long as several months.

Time-saving ideas

Obvious as it may be, organization is the key to staying on top of things with two babies. If you are bottle-feeding, you could make up twenty-four-hours' worth of milk in advance and store it in the fridge. Some mums use plastic formula travel containers to store pre-measured amounts of formula powder. These can be added more quickly to a bottle when a feed is made up. Try to wash and sterilize all your bottles at the same time of day, rather than doing them in dribs and drabs. Keep your changing bag stocked up with essentials to save having to check it at the last moment before you go out.

Are they identical and does it matter?

About one in three sets of twins are identical (monozygotic). These twins are formed from the same embryo and share the same DNA. The remainder are fraternal (dizygotic). They start as separate embryos, each with its own individual DNA and are no more alike than siblings.

While they are in the womb the majority of identical twins (about two thirds) will be monochorionic, which means they will be attached to the same placenta. An ultrasound scan can pick this information up quite easily and give instant confirmation that the twins are identical.

A minority of identical twins can cause confusion, though: they have di-chorionic, or separate, placentas, just as fraternal twins do. They are indistinguishable on an ultrasound scan from fraternal twins, which is why many hospitals misinform parents by telling them that their twins are definitely not identical when in fact they cannot be sure – unless one baby is a boy and the other a girl. If you have two placentas and your babies are the same sex they could be *either* identical or fraternal. If, once they arrive, it is not clear what they are, you can have their DNA tested very easily (see Notes, p. 290). (It isn't always immediately clear if twins are identical: there will always be slight differences between them, particularly differences of weight and size. Some parents have identical twins but insist they are not identical as they focus on the differences rather than the similarities.)

Knowing about their zygosity (as it's known) can be important if a medical condition arises with one twin. If the condition is genetic, it could arise with the other. It can also be helpful to know for sure when people question you, which they will. And it may strengthen your determination to treat your twins as individuals, and get others to do the same, if you know that they are identical. They themselves may also want to know – if not just yet – and find it strange if you do not.

Being identical could turn your twins into movie stars. Twins are highly sought after by television and film companies who get two interchangeable babies on set without anyone noticing. (There's some information in Notes on this.)

Feelings

> *'When I saw the two of them come out I thought "what a lot of work this is going to be" rather than "what darling little babies". They looked like a couple of little chickens and it was hard to feel any emotional attachment.*
>
> *'I did feel guilty about thinking that . . . but I think you should have an amnesty on guilt for the first six months . . .'*
> **Josh**

Bonding with twins is not always instantaneous. Being confronted by two frail-looking babies (as they often are) can make it hard to fall head over heels in love. The emotional attachment does of course come, but don't feel bad if at times you are as overwhelmed by the sheer hard work involved as you are by the joy of your babies' arrival. It may be many months before either parent feels the bonding process begin, but it will happen.

Some parents find that their babies' different personalities mean they react differently to each one, and feel guilty about doing so. For example, one baby may be more demanding than the other (and the babies may even reverse roles every few weeks). It's easy to fall into the habit of responding to the more vociferous baby and leaving the more placid one alone, sending a clear message that the way to get attention is to be outspoken. And there is the perpetual worry about whether your affections and attentions are being handed out in equal portions.

> *'In the beginning my little boy was much smaller and frailer: I was very worried and found myself drawn to him. I knew Gemma was fine but Tom looked so helpless and I probably "favoured" him in terms of attention. Even now I find that if either is sick, unwell or seems to be behind in*

any way I focus on that one. It all balances out in the end, but I do still beat myself up over whether I am giving each twin enough or equal attention.'
Cathy

Twin parents often find that the biggest pressure they face is on their own relationship, and recent research suggests fathers have a significant chance of developing depression. Postnatal depression is more prevalent among mothers of twins than for singleton babies (more so than for mothers of closely spaced singletons) and research among mums of twins under five shows that long-term depression is more likely as well (possibly the result of enduring exhaustion). Mothers of IVF twins may also be more vulnerable, finding themselves with what they (and everyone else) perceive as the answer to all their dreams and consequently unable to admit that the reality can be tougher than they had imagined.

None of this is meant to alarm you and it doesn't mean that if you have twins you will suffer from PND, but it probably does mean you owe it to yourself and your babies to seek advice if you have any reason to suspect you might be suffering from it (see p. 212 for more information).

Even if you don't get postnatal depression you may find yourself at a very low ebb a couple of weeks after your twins are born. Talking to another twin mum about how you feel may be all you need to realize that this is not abnormal and that it will pass. Here again your twins club should be invaluable. Someone in the club will be ready to offer a sympathetic and understanding ear. You may find that the people you meet there become friends whose support, as you embark on a lifetime as a twin or triplet parent, you will appreciate for many years.

Having twins is special; and whatever the increased worries, strains and pressures it can impose, few parents regret the experience. It's a cliché but 'double trouble' can also mean double the cuddles, double the fun and double the reward.

What if . . .

I am feeding my twins separately as I have no one to help me and they are still very tiny: they only weigh 6lb. How do I follow the routines while I do this?

Try to feed the babies as closely together as you can, waking one up as soon as the other has finished feeding. While they are still small you should limit each baby's feeds to half an hour; any more and the baby will be exhausted. This should mean you can get both feeds done within an hour. You will soon feel confident enough to feed both together.

I seem to be feeding my twins constantly and only have half an hour between one feed finishing and the next one starting. They are 11lb now.

Once you are feeding your babies at the same time things will get easier, and if your babies are 11lb they should be strong enough to be fed together, whether you are breast- or bottle-feeding. Remember not to let a feed last longer than an hour at the very most or both you and your babies will be exhausted.

My babies find it really difficult to latch on as they are small and sleepy. Should I persevere?

Wait until your babies are hungry before trying to get them to latch on. This will make them more likely to open their mouths wide, which is what they need to do to latch on. Waking a baby a quarter of an hour before a feed is important, especially when a baby is small and sleepy. It allows him to wake slowly and be ready to feed. Once his nappy is changed, he can be popped on a playmat or under an activity arch while you wait until he is ready to drink.

Set yourself a deadline for how long you are going to persist in trying to get your babies to take the breast. You could try for fifteen minutes, and if this doesn't work switch to feeding expressed milk from a bottle. It can be very distressing and exhausting for you to have a baby (or babies) who won't latch on, as well as frustrating for your baby (or babies). Setting yourself a time limit should reduce everyone's stress.

Remember to express regularly to keep up your milk supply.

When babies are small and sleepy it is really important that you do wake them for their feeds. Too often parents leave them to sleep during the day – for obvious reasons. They then have a difficult night when the babies wake from hunger because they have not drunk enough during the day. You must stick to the routine feed times.

When my twins came home from the Special Care Baby Unit they weighed 6lb and were on a four-hourly routine which I have stuck to. But four weeks later they are 9lb and they scream for their milk for half an hour before they are due to be fed.

When your babies were small and sleepy they were probably happy on a four-hourly routine, but they have now become more alert. A baby of 9lb should be fed more often than four-hourly so the best thing you can do is put them on a three- or three-and-a-half-hourly routine for a few weeks. You will not only find that this will make them happier during the day, it should also mean that they will be on course to sleep through the night as soon as they can because they will be getting more milk during the day and will be less likely to wake up through hunger at night.

I find it really hard to wind one baby while the other is still feeding. What can I do?

If you are breastfeeding, winding a baby over your shoulder is often the easiest method. Or lie one baby face-down across your knee. Keep lots of pillows within easy reach. You may have to stop feeding both babies to wind one while the other has a dummy.

One of my twins wakes the other one at night, even though they're in separate cots.
Most twins quickly get used to the presence of the other and sleep through their cries. Parents' fear that this won't happen can lead them to separate their twins, or to take one baby out of earshot of the other as soon as he cries. In fact, exposing twins to each other's noises may be the best way of ensuring that they do sleep through them. However, if yours persist in waking each other try putting them in separate rooms (if you can) until they are sleeping better.

My twins won't sleep at the same time.
If you keep feeding your twins at the same time and putting them down to sleep at the same time, they will eventually slip into a pattern of sleeping at the same time. Until they do, avoid the temptation to give in: unsynchronized twins are to be avoided.

13.

Finding Help for You and Your Baby

'Having a baby is hard work. In the first few days or weeks after your baby is born there will be times when you will feel exhausted, physically and emotionally. Just when you think you can grab an hour's sleep to recharge your batteries, you realize there is a pile of dirty washing in the corner and nothing to eat in the fridge.

'Asking for help, if you feel you need it, is nothing to be ashamed of. Nor is getting paid help – if you can afford it. Anything that eases the pressure and preserves your energy is good for both you and your baby.

'This chapter gives you some ideas on how you might get help, from family and friends to specialized babycare, some of it for the short term (postnatally) and some for longer. There are also some thoughts on how to make all of these work best for you.'

Barbara and Jo

Unpaid help

Friends

Friends can be strange when a new baby arrives. Some will bring you cooked meals or offer to do your shopping, while some will turn up uninvited and sit in your kitchen waiting to be served tea. Others may disappear altogether, terrified perhaps of babies, or of sleep-deprived fathers and hormonal mothers with whom conversation can be strained.

If you want to take your friends firmly in hand and get them to help out a little (without feeling too awkward about doing so), you might try a baby shower – but with a difference. With this type of baby shower you don't ask your friends for gifts. Instead you ask them to give you vouchers which are redeemable once your baby has arrived. The vouchers are for services, of your friends' choosing, and can be for as much or as little as they fancy. An evening's babysitting, a ready-cooked meal or a couple of hours of housework could be more useful to you than another set of babygros. It may seem a little brash, but some of your friends might actually prefer this option. You could even make the vouchers up yourself (ensuring that you get services that are actually going to be useful to you) and let your friends choose which ones they would like to give.

If this approach seems over-the-top, plan to have a list of chores that need doing and place it within easy view of all visitors. To avoid being the one who makes endless cups of tea once these friends have done their chores, stick notices on cupboard doors indicating where the tea, coffee, sugar and mugs are. With luck they will get the hint. Keeping a copy of your routine in a prominent place will also help them to know when they are most needed (feedtime perhaps) or best advised to leave (bedtime).

Don't expect friends to be knowledgeable about babycare, even if they are parents. It is easy to forget. You could get them simply to take your baby out for a walk, giving you a break to do whatever you want. If you have older children, explain to your friends how helpful it would be if they could lavish some attention on them at this time of change in their lives.

Friends with babies of their own may be too busy to help but may relish the idea of sharing babycare for short spells so each of you gets a break. Or you could exchange evening babysitting through a babysitting circle. Money need never change hands: instead use tokens in half-hour units for daytime babysitting and one-hour units for evening babysitting.

Family

Family members too can be strange when a new baby arrives. Older members may feel that their days of child-rearing are over and that you should cope on your own. Others may be desperate to help but not know whether they are wanted. You may need to reach out to them and say that their help would be gratefully received.

You could try asking your mother what *she* would most like to do to help with the baby. Not everyone finds it easy to have parents in their home. Talk about it with your partner and decide how you are going to manage any difficulties that may arise. You might agree to say yes to any help that parents offer, or you might think about setting some boundaries before your parents arrive, if you feel able to do that with them. It might make things run more smoothly. For example, you might feel that you are happy for them to take over the cooking but are not keen to be given too much advice on babycare. Tell them gently that you want to learn on your own, even if it means learning through your mistakes.

Whether family or friends, do try to space visitors. With a first baby you and your partner may want time alone in the first few days to get to know your baby. With subsequent babies you may want visitors as soon as possible to help with older children who are feeling left out.

Free help

If you need help badly (maybe you are unwell, called away for a family emergency or struggling alone with several children), but have no family or friends to rely on and paid help is not an option, you might be able to find a trainee nanny who will work for free. Childcare students often need work experience (see the twins chapter – trainees often favour families with twins but may also be interested in families with a newborn and a toddler). You cannot leave a student in sole charge of a baby but she should be able to help with any baby-related chores. Try your local training college or contact CACHE, the Council for Awards in Children's Care and Education.

Another place to look for help is the charity Home Start, which has volunteers who visit families needing support. The visits are free. Volunteers are not babysitters or cleaners, but they will stay with you for up to four hours, twice a week, and help in any way they can. If you think you are going to need help, it is worth enquiring about this service well in advance.

Your midwife is available to you for support and advice for twenty-eight days after the birth of your baby, and if you are struggling you should talk to her.

A health visitor will be on hand once your midwife's duties have ceased. She will know of local support groups for new mothers and if you are feeling isolated these can be really helpful. Sure Start areas (receiving government funding for services for children) sometimes offer occasional free places in crèches to help parents who need a break.

Paid help

Maternity nurses

If you've no idea what maternity nurses are, you're not alone. When you discover what they do to help new parents with their baby you might be tempted to find out more. But hold your fire until you find out how much they cost: this is the Rolls-Royce end of babycare options, both in terms of quality and price.

A maternity nurse can be a life-saver, or at least a sanity-saver, when you have a newborn. Put simply, her role is to move in with you as your guide and helper, armed with the knowledge you need to get your baby into a routine and in due course sleeping through the night. Should you have any concerns about your ability to achieve this on your own, you merely hand the task over to her.

Picture the scene: the nappy-bin has jammed; piles of unwashed laundry lie forlornly round the house; there is no food in the fridge; and before you stretches the certainty of another sleepless night soothing a screaming baby. Into this scene of chaos steps the maternity nurse – a modern Mary Poppins – bringing calm and order in her wake. Within minutes you and your baby are smiling and happy, a picture of contentment.

It isn't quite as simple as that, admittedly, but a maternity nurse can certainly cushion the shock of finding yourself under the same roof as a new baby, turning any stresses you may encounter into a happy and restful time. Her duties are extensive: she is responsible for helping parents with every aspect of caring for their baby, including bathing him, helping with all his feeds, settling him to sleep, and looking after him through the night. The baby's laundry is also her responsibility, as is sterilizing bottles and preparing formula, and she should keep his room clean and tidy and make sure he has the right equipment – a range of tasks requiring considerable organization skills.

She has responsibilities towards the mother, too, supporting her as she recovers from the birth and begins to breastfeed, and making sure that she eats, drinks and rests properly. She is *not* there to take over and look after the baby on her own – unless of course you want her to (and some parents do). Her role is to use her great expertise to help, teach and build parents' confidence.

And there's a bonus. Because a maternity nurse works through the night, you can catch up on your sleep if you want while she bottle-feeds your baby – with expressed breastmilk or formula. Or she can bring your baby to you when he's ready to be fed, and then settle him, however long it takes, while you go back to sleep. With luck, you'll be among the minority of new parents looking rested and relaxed, rather than haggard and tetchy.

A good maternity nurse should leave you feeling the money you spent on her, huge amount though it may be, was worth every penny – an investment for the whole family.

Who employs maternity nurses?

The rich and famous have nearly always had maternity nurses. But the not-so-rich – and not-at-all famous – now call on them too: new parents lacking confidence in dealing with a baby (especially if they have no family to help), older parents who doubt their ability to cope with sleepless nights, and mothers who have unexpectedly difficult births and need time to recover, or who simply find themselves in a fix and unable to cope (which is nothing to be ashamed of). Grandparents are even known to bestow the gift of a maternity nurse's services on their new grandchildren. Maternity nurses are particularly valued by parents having twins or triplets.

All these people have one thing in common: some spare cash. Maternity nurses fees start at around £450 a week, but are usually £600 or more, and up to £900/£1,000 a week for twins/triplets. (There's no tax or national insurance to pay on top as maternity nurses are self-employed.)

How much?! How long do they stay?

Most maternity nurses are booked to start a few days after a baby's due date and will stay for anything from two to eight weeks. For twins (or more) it's longer, usually six to twelve weeks. Some parents, though, find that a couple of weeks is enough to learn the ropes, get some sleep and then get on with the job on their own. Whether it's two weeks or twelve you have every right to get value for your money, which is why time spent looking for a maternity nurse who suits you, is so important.

Your search will be easier the earlier you start. Many of the best maternity nurses are booked up months in advance; some claim to get bookings on the day a pregnancy is confirmed. But even last-minute emergency bookings are nearly always possible.

How do I find a good maternity nurse?

One childcare book suggests maternity nurses come in two types: the old and experienced, and the young and inexperienced. This is simply not true. The two types of maternity nurse you'll find are the good ones ... and the not so good ones. Don't underestimate how important it is to find one of the former, but with demand outstripping supply they are much sought after.

Maternity nurses aren't necessarily qualified nurses at all, whatever their title may suggest. They don't have to have any formal training or any qualifications whatsoever. Some are former nurses or midwives and many are qualified nannies with a huge amount of experience with newborns; some have simply been doing the job for years. You will have to decide how important childcare qualifications are to you. This may matter more if you are expecting twins or triplets, who will be likely to have low birthweights and may need expert care.

There is no official register of maternity nurses as there is, for example, of childminders. This is surprising given the level of responsibility their job entails. Without a registering body to set standards and to record complaints of bad practice (which could lead to a member being struck off) it's impossible to guarantee that a maternity nurse has an unblemished record. So you may feel more comfortable using an agency – and you must ensure it is reputable. Qualifications, experience and references should be checked very carefully and you need some guarantee that the agency will do this thoroughly. The bottom line though is that if you have any worries you should double-check all references yourself.

What to ask when checking references

Picture yourself with a maternity nurse living in your house. You haven't liked her and don't want to recommend her to anyone else, but a few days before she's due to leave, she asks you to write a reference. You fear that telling the truth may turn things sour while she is still under your roof and with your baby in her care. The temptation to write a good reference for the sake of peace and harmony is great. And it happens.

Don't trust what is written on paper. References can lie.

The only way to establish the truth is to speak to the people who wrote them. Call the referees. Ask them whether the maternity nurse was easy to live with. If a routine and establishing good sleep habits are important to you, ask them whether she achieved this for their baby. Ask what they liked about her and what they didn't. Ask whether they still keep in touch.

If you ask just one question, ask whether they would employ her again.

The reason it's worth being thorough

In case you are not yet convinced of the need to be thorough, take note that the best of the breed are fantastic but the bad ones can spell disaster.

'I think a good maternity nurse should be planning her own redundancy from her job while she is with you. She should make sure that by the time she leaves, you don't need her because she has taught you how to thrive happily on your own. Sadly, it was we who were planning our maternity nurse's redundancy as I felt completely disempowered by her. She was so busy showing off her skills with babies that she never actually helped me, and never told me what to do when she left. As a result we were still feeding the boys four-hourly round the clock when they were six months old because we didn't know any better. By then we were so exhausted that we got another maternity nurse in to help. She had the boys sleeping through the night within a week. It transformed our lives.'
Katherine

'Although I wanted to get my twins into a routine, they were premature and needed to get their weights up first. But Phyllis insisted they should not be fed at night or they would never learn to sleep through. We believed she must know what she was doing but the health visitor discovered the babies were losing weight and were too small to be stretched to sleep through.

'Phyllis was putting their health at risk so we had no choice but to sack her. We discovered later that other families had had similar problems with her.'
Mary

What to ask a maternity nurse at interview

Don't underestimate how important the interview is. References are essential, but personality counts for a lot too: this is someone with whom you will be having an extremely close relationship. The interview is also your chance to double-check that you are getting what you want, especially if there is something that really matters to you. You'll kick yourself later if it turns out you weren't thorough enough.

Here's a checklist of things you could ask.

- Will she get your baby into a routine? Will she work towards getting him to sleep through the night and how will she achieve this? If she doesn't have a plan you may wonder what you are going to be paying for.
- Will she sleep in the baby's room if you want her to, and is she happy with the accommodation? If she says it's not good enough (and some maternity nurses can be very fussy), then find someone else.
- If you want to have time on your own with your baby, will she use that time to do other things such as playing with older siblings? (Some maternity nurses won't help you with anything but your new baby.)
- Will she be happy to take some direction from you or will you (or she) want her to take full charge?
- Will she take care of the night feed alone if you want her to?
- Is she willing to take her days off when it suits you?
- Will she be flexible about her duties, especially if things change unexpectedly and you have to travel, for example?
- If you don't breastfeed will she be supportive? You don't want a maternity nurse who tut-tuts in disapproval.
- Finally . . . if breastfeeding is important to you, will she encourage you? Ask her how she would help you to build your milk supply, or what she would advise if you ran into problems. In the event that you do encounter breastfeeding problems this sort of help is worth its weight in gold, but not all maternity nurses are good at helping a mum who is struggling with breastfeeding.

It may sound like hard work to go through all these points but it will pay off.

> 'Without my maternity nurse I wouldn't have kept up breastfeeding for one week, let alone the year that I eventually did. She made me believe I could do it, encouraging me to persevere when the going got tough. It would have been a lot easier for her to give in to the bottle. I can't thank her enough.'
> **Joanne**

Advice for parents on making things go smoothly

It may be helpful to sit down with a maternity nurse at the beginning of her stint with you and discuss what lies ahead. If you don't like something she suggests, say so now. You might also want to agree a time for a weekly informal chat when any problems can be raised openly and without awkwardness.

If there are other things that worry you, don't be embarrassed to raise them. This is a very special time for you and you need to enjoy it. Feel free to tell her that you need time on your own and when you would like it, and talk to her about what you want her to do when visitors arrive. If you don't want her to be around then say so.

It's also useful to agree between you when she can catch up on sleep. Although she's working for you twenty-four hours a day, she will need some time to sleep if the nights are difficult and it's best done at a time that is mutually agreed.

If all this advice fails and things go wrong it can feel catastrophic. Put it down to experience, part company and move on. Don't stick with it if it's not working because having a maternity nurse is only worthwhile if you and your baby end up happy.

'By the time my daughter was three weeks old I was struggling and decided to find a maternity nurse to help me. Esame was my life-saver. She arrived with her slippers in a bag, a smile on her face and I felt I had known her for ages. I managed to laugh for the first time since Harriet was born.

'She didn't tell me what to do, or how I should feel, or judge anything I was doing, but she showed me how to feed Harriet, how to get her into a routine, when she should sleep, how to wind her, bath her, play with her and most importantly she gave me the confidence to relax and enjoy my new baby.

'She stayed for about two weeks. It cost me £1,500 but was worth ten times that. I could catch up on sleep, allow my body to recover from the trauma of a difficult birth and I could hear my baby crying without fear or anxiety.

'If I have another baby I'm going to book Esame straight away.'
Julia

Alternatives to maternity nurses

If you can't afford a maternity nurse or don't want someone living in your house full time, but you do want experienced help, there are other options.

You could try to find a maternity trainee, a maternity nurse who will work for a reduced fee in order to gain extra experience. She should have some experience of babies already and be able to help you with night feeds and routine, all at about two-thirds of the price of her more experienced counterpart.

Night nannies for newborn babies are a relatively recent idea, and although a night nanny may not have the specialist experience of a maternity nurse, she can allow you the luxury of an occasional (or regular) night's sleep. If you want someone specifically to work on getting your baby to sleep through the night though, look for a night nanny who has a clear plan for doing this as not all of them do.

For specialized daytime help only you could try a maternity nanny, essentially a maternity nurse who doesn't do the night-shift. She will cost a little more than a regular nanny but will have more experience of newborn babies and can be hired for a fixed term.

Doulas

Doulas are an idea imported recently from the United States. (The Greek word means woman servant, or caregiver.) Birth doulas help parents before and during the birth (see p. 25) and postnatal doulas help parents afterwards. Some double up for both roles.

A postnatal doula's job is to care for a new mum. This is anything the mother wants, whether it be cleaning, cooking, running errands, doing the shopping or helping with basic baby-care, although most doulas do not have childcare qualifications. Their priority is the mother.

Doulas can usually offer flexible hours to suit your requirements and stay with you for anything from two to eight weeks.

'After my baby was born I wanted to look after him myself but I felt I needed someone to look after me. So I hired a doula. She did everything my mum would have done had she been around. She cooked, cleaned, fed and changed the baby (when I wanted her to) and babysat when I went out to shop or when I slept. She did five days a week for three weeks and at the end of her time I felt I was managing on my own.'
Claire

Nannies

Many nannies have experience with newborns so if you want to employ one to help with an older child (or children) once your baby arrives you might want one who can lend a hand with your baby too. Looking longer-term, nannies are usually the most flexible of childcare options, although that flexibility comes at a cost, which may be the reason that relatively few families go down this route. Salaries are quoted net of tax and national insurance which you the employer will have to pay.

A nanny's formal qualifications should include training in baby- and childcare, but if you find someone with no qualifications but many years of experience, don't rule them out.

Agency fees are steep so the least you should expect if you use one is that it makes a genuine effort to match you with a suitable candidate. As this does not always happen it is worth pursuing recommendations on agencies before choosing one. This also applies to agencies placing maternity nurses, doulas, mother's helps and au pairs. Unfortunately this is an industry which has acquired a reputation for allowing unreliable operators to flourish, but recent legislation has tightened up the regulation governing agencies placing childcarers and they are now subject to harsh penalties for malpractice. Agencies who belong to the Recruitment and Employment Confederation (a trade body for the recruitment industry) agree to abide by a code of practice.

And for even greater peace of mind it is always advisable to double-check references yourself. If you don't want to pay agency fees you will have to do this anyway. Finding a nanny independently has been made easy – certainly in the big cities – by the boom in childcare search sites on the web. If you don't live in a big city you can try advertising in local shops, newspapers or nurseries. Although it is more time-consuming to do the search yourself, don't assume you won't find someone as good as you might through an agency. You probably will.

If your nanny requirements are part-time you might look into sharing a nanny with another family, either splitting the nanny's week between you or getting her to look after your and their children at the same time.

Mother's helps

A mother's help may be an unqualified nanny, a nanny with limited experience of childcare, or simply a local woman who's good at helping out with housework and children. She is unlikely to be experienced with newborns and she may not be up to taking sole charge of a baby.

Her job is to help parents around the house, whether it be cleaning, cooking or shopping, as well as some basic childcare and help with older children if you have them. A mother's help will work similar hours to a nanny but will cost a little less, and this could be an ideal option if you work part-time or from home. Agencies supply mother's helps but again the fees are steep. The advice above on checking references is important here too.

Au pairs

The great thing about au pairs is that they are (relatively) inexpensive, partly because they always live in. And because they are not officially classed as employees you don't have to pay their national insurance or tax. The downside is that they are also (relatively) inexperienced so are unlikely to be much help with a baby. But a good one could lighten your load by doing some housework and cooking, or entertaining older children.

Given that an au pair is in the country to learn the language and culture, needs time off to study, and may not speak great

English you might feel this is too much of a hassle. An au pair will usually hope to stay in a family for at least six months. If in that time you go back to work she will not be the solution to childcare.

As well as agencies, there are websites specializing in placing au pairs. Many au pairs are based in their home country and cannot be met beforehand for an interview. The risk is yours.

What to ask referees

With doulas, mother's helps, nannies and au pairs – as with maternity nurses (see above) – remember that written references can lie. You need to check them. Many is the parent who has given a pleasant reference for an outgoing carer as a way of ending a relationship on good terms. If you ask a referee nothing else, ask about the childcarer's strengths, time-keeping, sickness record and any areas that former employers were unhappy about. It may be that someone with great strengths had a major weakness that a former employer needs prompting to mention.

Find out from the referee why their childcarer left and always ask whether they would employ her again. This can be the most revealing question: if you notice any hesitation, think twice before offering the job.

Childminders

This is a very popular choice for working parents (particularly for very young children) partly because it is one of the most afford-able. Childminders charge by either the hour or the day and, although costs vary considerably, are around £120 per week (five full days) per child.

Childminders look after your baby from about the age of six weeks in their homes, although some will come to you and take care of him in your own home. They can even continue to look after your child once he reaches school age, during out-of-school hours.

Childminders are registered with the government body Ofsted, the Office for Standards in Education, which means they will have passed police checks and be subject to Ofsted inspections every two years, as well as regulations on how many children they can care for at a time. Childminders do not have to have any formal childcare qualifications, so it's up to you to assess how suitable a particular childminder would be for your child.

Your local Children's Information Service will have full details of all the childminders in your area.

Day nurseries

This is a booming business that has expanded rapidly in recent years, and the majority of day nurseries are privately owned. Costs will usually be higher than for childminders and range from about £130 to £200 for a full-time place, although prices in inner London may be as high as £300. Most nurseries take babies from fifteen weeks and they differ from pre-school nurseries in that they cater specifically for working parents, being open from around 8 a.m. to 6 p.m., fifty or so weeks a year. They have to be registered with Ofsted, have a minimum number of trained staff, and are subject to regulations on the ratio of children to adults. Ofsted officers visit nurseries regularly to carry out inspections.

State help with childcare

In addition to the universal Child Benefit (but claim it as soon as you can after your child is born because if you delay you may lose some benefit), low-income working families are entitled to tax credits for childcare. This includes childminders but not nannies (although this is changing – under a new scheme for accredited nannies). Free nursery (pre-school) education is not available until your child is three years old unless he has special needs.

Whatever form of childcare you choose, whether it be a maternity nurse or nursery, it is worth remembering that if things don't work out, it's best for everyone if you act immediately to sort the problem. This may seem daunting if you are working full-time and fear you won't find a replacement fast enough, but there are few things as stressful as having unsatisfactory childcare. Parents always say how relieved they are that they acted, rather than sat on the problem.

14.
Other Secrets

'Watching my nephew Hadleigh react to the arrival of his baby sister, Freya, made me realize the truth of what I have been telling parents for years. Having a baby on a routine is good not just for the baby and for the parents, it is good for older brothers and sisters too.

'Hadleigh had been a difficult baby with a dairy intolerance and was a poor sleeper. He never strictly followed one of my routines and didn't sleep through the night until he was one year old. When Freya was born my sister Nic had no hesitation in putting her on a three-hourly routine and introducing a bedtime ritual at 7 p.m. She was settling within days and sleeping through the night at twelve weeks.

'My sister was thrilled . . . not just about Freya but also about the effect this had on Hadleigh. During the day he knew when mum was going to have time for him. He also knew that as the "big boy" he got to go to bed later and have mum and dad all to himself from seven to eight o'clock in the evening. Nic was amazed by how loving he was to Freya as a result. She was also amazed at how Freya's routine meant she could get Freya and Hadleigh up, dressed and ready to leave the house for Hadleigh's playgroup by 9 a.m. every day.

'This chapter will give you some ideas on preparing for the arrival of a sibling, as well as guidance on travelling with a routine, and finally on going back to work.'

Jo

Siblings

It may seem obvious but research has been conducted to prove it: children who are most upset by a new arrival are those who experience the most dramatic drop in parental attention. But how do you get round that problem?

This is where a routine for your new baby can be a boon. It will allow you to pre-plan the time you can devote to the older children and let them know this in advance, rather than leaving it to chance, which can be very frustrating for young kids. There is also the added bonus to everyone of having a baby who sleeps through the night at an early age. In fact, some parents find that having a routine for a second or subsequent baby is the only way they can keep things on track.

If you know that your older child's established routines will clash with your baby's, try to make changes before the baby arrives. If that proves difficult, remember to make the most of the flexibility of the routines when you need to. Just follow the order of events – wake, feed, play and nap – and choose a bedtime for your baby that you know you can stick to consistently.

It is easier for a new baby to learn his bedtime ritual and settling routine if older siblings aren't around to interrupt. If they insist on watching, or if you have no way of entertaining them while you settle the baby, tell them they can watch if they sit by the door and don't talk.

Here are a few other ideas for easing the transition for your older child or children.

Preparing a big brother or sister for a new baby

Getting older kids as involved as possible in the build-up to the birth is helpful, but timing it right may be hard as a young child may get impatient if he has to wait several months for a baby's arrival.

As you prepare your new baby's cot try to include your older child: get him to help choose and sort clothes or toys. One parent wished she had got her son to make the decisions about which of his toys he wanted to pass on to his baby sister as he became possessive about them later on. Take him on a shopping trip just before the baby is due and get him to choose some presents for his new brother or sister. Buy some presents from the new baby for him.

Keep reminding your child how much you love him and explain that you have enough love for him as well as the new baby; if he is your first, you might like to explain that he will always be your first and will always be special. Look at photos or videos of him as a baby and talk about what he was like. Keep talking about the baby and involve him in choosing a name. If you haven't got one, you could give the baby a nickname.

> 'Calling the baby "Felix" during my pregnancy really helped Billy and Jessie to understand that mummy had a baby in her tummy and that Felix would be part of the family. I would ask them what they would say to the baby when he arrived and they would reply "Hello Felix". Once Joseph was born we explained that Felix now had a new name. We had no jealousy problems even though Billy and Jessie were two and a half and eighteen months, so maybe this helped.'
> **Mary**

Once the baby arrives

Your baby's arrival in his new home is a very special event. To make it a little easier for an older child, you could get someone other than mum (a neighbour or grandparent) to bring your new baby into the house while you are with your firstborn. You could then spend time with him before asking him to help you to introduce the baby to the home.

Once you are home your older child will probably test you, so try to do exactly as you did before. Acting up often happens when mum is breastfeeding because it is harder for her to respond. Try to nip this in the bud: stop feeding your baby and deal with the problem or it may be repeated. Don't be tempted to give up on discipline. Siblings will often try to hurt a new baby so decide what you are going to do about this and be consistent. If you are worried about your baby being hurt when your back is turned, put him in his rocker chair inside a playpen to be on the safe side. Whenever you see your older child getting irritable or annoyed with the baby it's best to separate them.

Reward your older child every time he is nice to the baby and tell him often, and emphatically, that the new baby likes him. You could pretend the baby can speak, and put words into his mouth, saying nice things to his older brother or sister.

Do explain that it will take a long time for the baby to be doing things as children can get very excited by the idea that mummy is going to bring them a brother or sister, and then be frustrated when the baby arrives and can't play. Tell your older child that babies cry a lot and can be very smelly. He will find the baby interesting if you talk about him. Use positive terms if you can: try not to say 'don't touch the baby's eyes' but rather 'the baby's eyes are very delicate; try touching his cheek'. Keeping physical contact – including hugs and kisses – short will limit how often you have to intervene.

Remind your older child of how many things he can do that the baby can't. Being 'mummy's little helper' makes older siblings feel important. But don't rely on the help too much. One four-year-old, when asked to fetch one too many nappies for her mother, said, 'Not again! You're the mummy, it's your job.'

A toddler who normally sleeps well may be woken by a new

baby's cries. If this happens, put him back to bed as quickly as you can and with a minimum of fuss so a habit doesn't set in. It will take him time to get used to the new baby's cries but if he has slept well in the past he will do so again and will sleep through the noise.

A first-born may need a year to adjust to a new baby brother or sister; as he gets used to one phase the baby moves on to another and he has to adapt again. Don't be alarmed if he regresses to wanting to use a potty or waking up at night for no apparent reason. It is usually just a phase.

Sometimes the hardest thing for parents, when they're so excited about their new baby, is to acknowledge that their older child has negative feelings. But it can be really helpful if parents acknowledge those feelings because blocking them can lead to the simultaneous blocking of positive feelings. If you see that your older child is upset try to talk to him, but away from the baby. Ask him to tell you if he feels cross. The more you can accept – and let him know that you accept – that his feelings are normal, the more it will help him come to terms with them.

'When talking to parents expecting a second or third child I remind them that children notice a lot more than they might think and I tell them one of my favourite stories. One mum I knew was having a hard time getting her five-year-old, two-year-old and new baby into the car and shouted "Be quiet". Silence. Then a little voice piped up, "You can't cope with three children, can you mummy?" To which the mother replied, "Yes, I can, but not you three!"'

Jo

What if there are two?

The arrival of twins can be particularly tough for an older child, and with your hands doubly full you will have little time to help him as much as you might like. Despite your best efforts, well-meaning friends and even strangers will often focus on the twins and leave their big brother or sister in the shade. Shifting everyone's focus to your older child is key but not easy.

> 'Lachlan was two when his twin sisters arrived and too young to express his feelings. But my feelings were so much stronger for the child I knew versus the new additions that I was obsessed with how to make it easier on him. We made sure that he got some serious time with us on our own, even in the first few days home from hospital. It was hard at times to do things when I really wanted to take a few minutes' break or sleep but I am glad I stayed focused on him.
>
> 'Much later, when he was three, Lachlan had a series of tantrums that made our heads spin: looking back it was probably to be expected he would eventually react. Luckily we were able again to arrange for him to have time with me on his own and all is now back on track a year later. We have conditioned ourselves to have absolutely no guilt in taking him out to lunch or a movie without his sisters. He gets more one-on-one time with his parents than he ever would have if we'd only had one second child and my only regret is that we can't provide the same for the girls because they are twins.'
> **Jacki**

Travel

'Once my boys were settled into their routine, I thought that travelling would be out. I couldn't have been more wrong. I came to discover that the joy of routines is that they work wherever you go. The key is to stick to feeding and nap times as closely as you can, whether you are going away for a few days or a few hours. It can take a bit of planning but the routine helps a baby feel at home in a strange place. Once I realized this, I felt comfortable taking the boys anywhere and everywhere.'
Barbara

Imagine you're on the motorway and it's time for your baby to feed. You might start cursing your routine. But all you need to do is plan ahead of your journey to be somewhere you can feed when the time comes (even a motorway service station). That's much easier than being caught unawares by a starving baby when you're in the fast lane and twenty miles from a turn-off.

Plan stops on your journey when your baby can get out of the car and have a change of scenery. He will get bored after a while sitting in a car seat and even a service station car park will seem interesting. The motion of the car may lull him into long sleeps, but it is unlikely that this will impact much on his night-time sleep, so don't be tempted to keep him up later than his usual bedtime when you arrive at your destination, in the hope that he will sleep better. He may get overtired and sleep worse.

A big event, such as a wedding, is nothing to worry about. You could rearrange things so you feed your baby before the service. Then he'll either sleep through it or gurgle contentedly with a full tummy. Carry a dummy for any quiet moments in the service, and if you take him to the reception make sure he isn't passed around like a parcel or he'll get fractious. Pop him in his pushchair when you feel the time is right so he can have some quiet time in a corner without the distraction of faces and bright lights.

When you stay away overnight just re-create what you do at home at bedtime. Take a couple of your baby's favourite cuddly toys and if he has a lullaby soother take that too and pack his cot mobile for the mornings. Try to make the new bedroom as dark as possible. Take a length of blackout material or a black dustbin bag, some bulldog clips, sticky tape or pins and stick it over the window in the room where your baby is sleeping.

Then follow your bedtime ritual as near as possible to the time that you do it at home. Ignore unhelpful comments from friends such as 'Can't you keep the baby up later so we can play with him?' A baby who has a consistent bedtime ritual will amaze you by his adaptability to new surroundings. Follow the sequence of events of your ritual from his bath to his feed to putting him down awake. Say goodnight and leave.

If you want to take your baby to the evening reception (and this can also apply if at any time you want to go out in the evening and cannot find anyone to babysit), follow the bedtime ritual, then swaddle your baby (if he's still young enough to be swaddled) and put him in his pram or pushchair. Take a dark sheet or blanket to drape over the pram to block out any bright lights and take him with you. He should settle just as he does at home. If he doesn't, rock the pram and soothe him for a bit to help him. Try to be back in time for the late-night feed, after which you can put him in his cot for the night.

When you are away treat the night-time feeds as you would at home, using spaced soothing when you need to. Parents understandably worry that other people will be disturbed by their baby's cries and sometimes deviate from the routine they're in. But this can have consequences . . .

One mum and dad took their eight-week-old daughter to

friends in the country and she started to wake at 5.30 because her room was light. Her parents, worried that she would disturb everyone else, got her up, dressed her and started to play. When they returned home she carried on waking at 5.30 because she now assumed someone would come and play.

If your journey involves changing time zones, follow the routine times until you arrive at your destination. Then switch the timings to match the new time zone the minute you arrive.

Here are a few other tips that might be helpful.

Planes

Airlines are legally obliged to provide you with a separate seat belt for your baby; this attaches to your own while you hold your baby on your lap. During take-off and landing, babies' ears can be sensitive so take a dummy and wiggle it in your baby's mouth to make him suck, which should take some of the pressure off his ears. Or try giving him a bottle of cooled boiled water to suck on.

For ease (if you are bottle-feeding) take disposable bottles or a travel system with pre-sterilized bags that you simply throw away. For further ease use pre-made carton milk. If your baby has been weaned, don't rely on the airline to provide anything suitable to eat.

Buy lots of small, cheap and cheerful toys to entertain your little one. You can swap them as soon as he gets bored, lose them without worrying too much, and throw them away at the end of your trip.

Hire cars

If you are hiring a car order a baby seat in advance so that you can be sure the company will supply one. It isn't always guaranteed, so if you're worried it may be safest to take your own.

Will people glare at me if my baby cries on the plane/train?

Of course they will. But it's part and parcel of life as a parent. If disapproving stares worry you, avoid eye contact with other travellers. Shrug off silly comments, and remember that everyone was a baby once. If you have the nerve, beam at everyone around you with parental pride. Who knows – if your baby makes enough noise, you might find that all the nearby seats are vacated and you have more room than you could have hoped for.

What happens when the clocks change?

Try changing the times of your baby's routine by fifteen minutes for each of the two days preceding the clock change. Once it happens you will then be only half an hour out of sync. Follow the new time straight away and you should find your baby slips into it without a murmur.

Returning to work

> 'My boss thought I was exactly the same person as the one he remembered before I left for maternity leave. But I wasn't. The job had moved on while I was away and I was out of touch. I had to bite the bullet, sit him down and tell him that I needed time to readjust.'
> **Ann**

What's so hard about going back to work?

Looked at from the comparative calm of pregnancy it can seem as simple as finding and organizing suitable childcare. Now, with a baby smiling up at you from his cot, it can seem like an act of betrayal. Who can I really trust with my child? Am I being selfish to want to reclaim my old life? Will I still be able to do my job?

Although some women look forward to returning to work as quickly as possible, the majority do not. A recent survey found that 75 per cent of mothers-to-be said they would not return to work after their babies were born if their finances allowed it. So if you feel reluctant about going back, you are not alone. Perhaps it is an awareness of the enormous demands that a family and work can impose. The vast majority of working mothers questioned said they felt 'exhausted all the time' as well as guilty about being away from their children. Two thirds also said they worried about the cost of childcare, which is hardly surprising given that childcare in Britain is the most expensive in Europe.

If you want and can afford to work part-time, the law states that your employer must consider your request to work flexibly, but he does not have to agree to it. He does, however, have to prove that he has tried to accommodate your request and demonstrate his reasons for not granting it. While some employers are sympathetic to the needs of returning mums, others may leave you feeling that you are making unreasonable demands if full-time work no longer suits you. If yours is in the latter camp, don't let yourself be browbeaten. Only a quarter of women who go back to work in the first year after having a baby do so full-time.

If you are returning to work at the end of so-called ordinary maternity leave, you are entitled to the same job on the same conditions. If you return after additional maternity leave, you are entitled to the same job on the same conditions unless it is not reasonably practicable for your employer to take you back in your original job, in which case you have the right to be offered suitable alternative work. If you are due to return to work at the end of your maternity leave but cannot because you are ill, you should still be entitled to sick pay as long as you follow your employer's sickness procedures. This also applies if you have postnatal depression or other post-pregnancy illnesses.

Whatever you do and whenever you do it, having a routine for your baby will, again, help. If your baby is cared for at home when you return to work, you can ensure that his daily timetable continues as before, giving him continuity while you're away. And assuming he's sleeping at night you yourself will be better prepared for a working day.

> *'I went back to work five months after the birth of each of my girls. My nanny picked up the routine they were in and I felt happy knowing that although I wasn't with them, I knew exactly what they were doing practically to the half hour. My nanny found this helpful too and I think it gave the girls a sense of continuity.'*
> **Annabel**

Equally, if you place your baby in registered childcare the childcarer should be understanding about your routine and adapt to it, so your baby does not get confused.

Dads and work

> *'Going back to work was very, very strange. I realized I was missing my daughter and thinking about her all the time. Another person had entered my life. It was like a love affair.'*
> **Richard**

British dads are doing more and more childcare. In the mid-1970s, fathers spent less than a quarter of an hour a day on child-related activities; that figure has now risen to two hours a day. So, mums, you have nothing to complain about.

However, British men also work some of the longest hours in Europe. Which means that many dads are burning the candle at both ends, and that can cause strains – both at work and between partners. Fathers sometimes feel that the way they juggle their lives after a baby is born is obscured by the mother's presence at the centre of the baby's life. Dads too can undergo a change in their feelings about work once a baby has arrived, yet be unable to express those feelings for fear it seems they lack commitment to the job. Many employers still view flexible working as something for women alone, and men may feel reluctant to ask for it, although they are entitled to do so.

This is all said in the spirit of helping dads feel they are not alone. And for mums to remember that dads and their feelings at work count too.

Giving up breastfeeding

If you need to phase out your breastfeeding before returning to work there are ways of making the transition smooth. It takes up to two weeks to give up breastfeeding step by step, if it is not to be an uncomfortable or even painful process. (The exact length of time will depend on how well your baby sleeps at night and how many feeds you are doing when you stop.) After this time your breasts will continue to produce small quantities of milk for a while. (If you change your mind about giving up breastfeeding during this time you can probably still resume it. Give a breastfeed followed by a top-up of formula and decrease the amount of formula every few days. You could also express to boost your milk supply.)

Returning to work doesn't automatically mean you have to give up breastfeeding. You could take a breast pump to work and keep expressed milk in a fridge before taking it home. Or you could express and discard the milk simply to keep your milk supply high. Your employer is supposed to allow rest periods for this as well as a place to express and somewhere to store milk.

If you don't take to the idea of expressing in your office, one of the most successful ways of winding down your breastfeeding is to cut out one feed every three days until you are left with the morning and bedtime feeds. You could keep these going for a while or finish them last (add another six days to the plan below). These are often the most rewarding feeds for both mother and baby.

The first feeds to stop would obviously be the night-time ones. A bottle of formula may have the added benefit of helping a baby to sleep a little longer. However, some babies resist this as they can smell their mother's milk, so it may be that your partner has to take over at this point.

If your baby is already sleeping between 11 p.m. and 7 a.m., you will have only one night-time feed to switch, the 11 p.m. dream feed, so do this first. Then switch the feeds in the middle of the day, starting around three days later. If your baby is sleeping from 7 p.m. to 7 a.m. then this all becomes academic as you can start on the daytime plan straight away.

Below are two plans to follow to give up daytime breastfeeds gradually, based on the three-hourly and the four-hourly routine (you can adapt them if you are on any of the other routines), and leaving you with the option of continuing to breastfeed in the early morning and evening before and after work.

9-day plan: 3-hourly routine

Days 1–3

7 a.m.	Breastfeed.
10 a.m.	Formula feed replaces breastfeed.
1 p.m.	Breastfeed.
4 p.m.	Breastfeed.
7 p.m.	Breastfeed.
11 p.m.	Formula feed.

Days 4–6

7 a.m.   Breastfeed.
10 a.m. Formula feed replaces breastfeed.
1 p.m.   Breastfeed.
4 p.m.   Formula feed replaces breastfeed.
7 p.m.   Breastfeed.
11 p.m. Formula feed.

Days 7–9

7 a.m.   Breastfeed.
10 a.m. Formula feed replaces breastfeed.
1 p.m.   Formula feed replaces breastfeed.
4 p.m.   Formula feed replaces breastfeed.
7 p.m.   Breastfeed.
11 p.m. Formula feed.

6-day plan: 4-hourly routine

Days 1–3

7 a.m.   Breastfeed.
11 a.m. Formula feed replaces breastfeed.
3 p.m.   Breastfeed.
7 p.m.   Breastfeed.
11 p.m. Formula feed.

Days 4–6

7 a.m.	Breastfeed.
11 a.m.	Formula feed replaces breastfeed.
3 p.m.	Formula feed replaces breastfeed.
7 p.m.	Breastfeed.
11 p.m.	Formula feed.

If you cannot continue to feed in the mornings or evenings, cut these feeds out next, dropping one every three days.

A problem may arise if at first your baby hates formula, which tastes very different from breastmilk. Try giving him a bottle of formula and if he refuses give him a bottle of expressed breastmilk. Then try again at the next feed. Or feed your baby a mixture of formula and breastmilk, gradually increasing the proportion of formula. (If your baby is refusing a bottle altogether, see p. 129.) Whatever you decide to do, allow yourself time to achieve it.

'I thought that when I went back to work it would be easy to get Hadleigh on to bottles. How wrong I was! It was the night-time feeds that were difficult. Every time I offered him a bottle he screamed. The problem was that he could smell my milk. It got so bad that I ended up in tears. The only thing I could do was to get my husband to do the night feed. He wasn't thrilled but it worked and within days Hadleigh was taking a bottle at night.'
Nic

Notes

Here are some personal recommendations on where to source some of the equipment referred to in this book and where to find more information, help or advice. This list is by no means exhaustive.

1. The secret to being prepared

Nappies

For all you need to know about washable/cloth nappies there is an independent advice service called The Nappy Lady www.the nappylady.co.uk. Or email Marion Hope on www.marion@the nappylady.co.uk direct (one of the Nappy Lady's advisers and a friend of ours!). If you would like the dirty nappies taken away, cleaned and delivered back to you (London and some other areas) log on to www.nappyexpress.com.

If you need low-birthweight disposable nappies try Boots or Tesco.

Rocker chairs

These are sometimes known as bouncing chairs. Jo's favourites are the ones made by Chicco. They are well padded and recline flat.

Breast pumps/expressing machines

You can buy or hire electric breast pumps through the following two sites: www.ameda.demon.co.uk and www.breastpumps. co.uk/expression.htm – they usually deliver overnight. You may also be able to hire a breast pump through your local branch of the National Childbirth Trust, the NCT www.nctpregnancyand babycare.com.

Bottles

Both Tommee Tippee and Avent make wide-necked bottles. For latex teats try NUK orthodontic teats which come in two different sizes and three different thicknesses – they are sold at Superdrug, larger baby-feeding departments of Boots, and some small private pharmacies. They can also be bought online from: www.baby-supplies.co.uk or www.pharmacy2u.co.uk.

Toys

For black, white, red and boldy coloured toys for small babies try the 'Whoozit' baby range by Manhattan Baby, or Lamaze baby toys, all of which are available from baby equipment retailers.

Television

'Baby Mozart' is part of the American *Baby Einstein* range. There are others including a new range called 'Baby Bright', produced in association with the Great Ormond Street Hospital.

Slumber Bear

The Slumber Bear is made by Prince Lionheart, www.princelionheart.com. Or try a First Year's Lullaby Player or the Fisher Price Lullaby Soother.

Dummies/soothers

Avent make dummies with protective covers.

The calculation on parents' spending on their baby in the first year was by *Prima* magazine.

Buying second-hand/on the web

Many baby items can be bought second-hand on eBay: www.ebay.co.uk. www.ukparents.co.uk has a buy (and sell) forum. Try the National Childbirth Trust for local sales of second-hand maternity clothes, baby clothes, toys and equipment: www.nctpregnancyandbabycare.com. For twins-club sales of the same look at www.twinsclub.co.uk which carries notices of sales around the country. There are many Internet sites selling (new) baby equipment: www.kiddicare.com seems to be one of the top discounters, although its range is limited and all enquiries have to be by email.

To pick up tips from other mums you could try websites with message/chat boards for parents and parents-to-be, for example www.ukparents.co.uk.

2. Getting off to a flying start

Home births

Information and support is offered by the pressure group AIMS, the Association for Improvements in the Maternity Services www.aims.org.uk. AIMS publishes a booklet called *Choosing a Home Birth* which you might find helpful. They also have other publications on women's options during pregnancy and childbirth. You could also try BirthChoiceUK www.birthchoiceuk.com.

An independent midwife or doula

Contact the Independent Midwives Association for advice on how to hire an independent midwife www.independentmidwives.org.uk. If you want a birth doula, try www.doula.org.uk.

Birthing pools

These are available from: Splashdown Water Birth Services www.waterbirth.co.uk, Birthworks www.birthworks.co.uk and The Active Birth Centre www.active birthcentre.com.

Baby massage

You can read about the benefits of baby massage on the website of the Infant Massage Information Service at www.infantmassageimis.com.au and The International Association of Infant Massage at www.iaim.org.uk, where there are also recommended books showing in detail how to massage your baby.

Breastfeeding

The National Childbirth Trust helpline should be able to give you phone numbers for local breastfeeding support groups (0870 444 8708, 8 a.m.–10 p.m.) or you may be able to speak to one of their counsellors on the phone. Their website is at www.nctpregnancyandbabycare.com.

You could also try the Breastfeeding Network Supporters line (0870 900 8787) or www.breastfeedingnetwork.org.uk. The BfN runs some drop-in centres where you can seek advice face to face.

To hire a private lactation consultant try the Lactation Consultants of Great Britain www.lcgb.org.uk or the International Lactation Consultant Association www.ilca.org.

It is worth remembering that when it comes to babies and breastfeeding, there are strongly held views about the choice between routine- and demand-feeding. If, when you seek advice, you encounter opposition to what you are doing, please remember that the decision is yours and yours alone. It is not someone else's.

Safeguarding against cot death

The Foundation for the Study of Infant Deaths (Sudden Infant Death Syndrome) has full and detailed advice on reducing the risk of cot death at www.sids.org.uk.

Research showing the benefits of swaddling babies was done in the USA at the Washington University School of Medicine.

11. Minor ailments and upsets

Cranial osteopathy

If you want to consult a cranial osteopath, try The Sutherland Society (the UK Organisation for Cranial Osteopathy), www.cranial.org.uk.

The two studies on cranial osteopathy and its effect on babies are 'Towards an Understanding of Osteopathy in the Treatment of Infantile Colic' by C. J. Hayden (published in the *Journal of Manual & Manipulative Therapy*, 2002) and 'A Study of the Efficacy of Cranial Osteopathic Treatment on Neonates, Infants and Children with Sleep Disturbances' by Philip Owen (you can read it at www.childrens clinic.co.uk).

Postnatal depression

For information on postnatal depression try The Association for Postnatal Illness www.apni.org.uk

Getting back into shape

For more information on Pilates contact Pilates and yoga teacher Melissa Cosby at melissa.pilates@mac.com

12. Twin secrets

For information on the Multiple Births Foundation evenings for parents expecting multiples, check the MBF's website www.multiplebirths.org.uk. The MBF can also give you information on zygosity testing (a DNA test to determine whether twins or triplets are identical).

To find your local twins club, and to join Tamba, see the website of the Twins and Multiple Births Association at www.tamba.org.uk. Tamba's freephone helpline, Twinline, is 0800 138 0509.

To pick up tips from other mums of, or expecting, multiples try the message/ chat boards at www.tamba.org.uk or www.twinsclub.co.uk.

You can find twin nursing pillows, Podee bottles and stroller connectors at www.jusonneuk.co.uk and www.2became4.com.

Mums of aspiring (identical) twin television stars might like to contact Karin Wayment (a mum of twins herself) at the agency Twins and Triplets. Babies in particular are in demand. You can email Karin via Twinsontv@aol.com.

Research on fathers of twins and depression conducted by Debbie Sen, Newcastle Twin Study, PhD work, Newcastle University.

13. Finding help for you and your baby

Free help

Childcare students who have reached a certain level in their studies may be placed in families with at least two children, generally with one child under three and one less than a year old. The idea is to give students hands-on experience but in the presence of a mother. The student must never be left alone with the children. CACHE, the Council for Awards in Children's Care and Education, www.cache.org.uk, is connected to 1,000 centres where childcare is studied and should be able to give you the names of colleges in your local area.

To find a Home Start volunteer try www.home-start.org.uk (08000 68 63 68).

Maternity nurses/nannies

If you are looking for a maternity nurse try The Maternity Nurse Company, which is based in Harrogate but places maternity nurses all round the country (01423 709679). The Maternity Nurse Company may also be able to place a (less expensive) maternity trainee if you want one.

Several nanny agencies now offer night nannies and maternity nannies.

If you don't want to use an agency to find a maternity nurse, nanny, doula or any other type of help with your baby you can either search CVs or place an advert in the following websites: www.thegumtree.com or www.nannyjob.co.uk. (But be warned – these sites tend to have a bias to the southeast of England.) Or try the publications *Simply Childcare* www.simplychildcare.com or *The Lady*.

Childminders and nurseries

You can get a list of childminders and nurseries from the Children's Information Service at your local authority or try online at www.childcarelink.gov.uk.

'Choosing Childcare: Your Sure Start guide to childcare and early education' is available free of charge from Daycare Trust through their helpline (020 7840 3350). It contains information and advice on the different childcare options available, what to look for in quality care and help on affording childcare.

14. Other secrets

The Maternity Alliance is a national charity (www.maternityalliance.org.uk) which, among other things, has comprehensive advice about maternity (and paternity) leave and returning to work. You could also try Working Families at www.working families.org.uk or the government website www.dti.gov.uk/workingparents.

Index